The Politics of Pain Medicine

The Politics of Pain Medicine

A Rhetorical-Ontological Inquiry

S. SCOTT GRAHAM

THE UNIVERSITY OF CHICAGO PRESS   CHICAGO AND LONDON

S. SCOTT GRAHAM is director of the Scientific and Medical Communications Laboratory and assistant professor in the English department at the University of Wisconsin–Milwaukee.

The University of Chicago Press, Chicago 60637
The University of Chicago Press, Ltd., London
© 2015 by The University of Chicago
All rights reserved. Published 2015.
Printed in the United States of America

24 23 22 21 20 19 18 17 16 15   1 2 3 4 5

ISBN-13: 978-0-226-26405-9 (cloth)
ISBN-13: 978-0-226-26419-6 (e-book)
DOI: 10.7208/chicago/9780226264196.001.0001

Library of Congress Cataloging-in-Publication Data

Graham, S. Scott, author.
  The politics of pain medicine: a rhetorical-ontological inquiry / S. Scott Graham.
      pages; cm
  Includes bibliographical references and index.
  ISBN 978-0-226-26405-9 (cloth: alk. paper) — ISBN 978-0-226-26419-6 (e-book)
1. Pain medicine. 2. Pain—Treatment. 3. Pain—Treatment—Psychological aspects.
4. Psychophysiology. 5. Medicine, Psychosomatic. 6. Midwest Pain Group.   I. Title.
  RB127.G726 2015
    616'.0472—dc23   2015001522

♾ This paper meets the requirements of ANSI/NISO Z39.48-1992 (Permanence of Paper).

Contents

Acknowledgments

Certainly a project like *The Politics of Pain Medicine* could not have come to fruition without a great deal of support, and I would be remiss if I didn't publicly acknowledge the many people who helped this work along the way. First, a project like this is simply not possible without the gift of access. I cannot offer enough thanks to the Midwest Pain Group, its members, and my other informants in the larger national pain management community. Without their willingness to participate and insightful discussions of the relationship between my work and theirs, this book would not exist.

Additionally, I have presented early versions of my inquiries into pain medicine and rhetorical-ontological methodologies at a variety of scholarly conferences, and I am especially grateful to the many members of the Association for the Rhetoric of Science and Technology, the Rhetoric Society of America, and the Association for Teachers of Technical Writing, whose thoughtful engagement with these early efforts contributed significantly to the final realization of this book. Furthermore, I was able to publish several early analyses of the Midwest Pain Group and pain-related pharmaceuticals policy in the *Technical Communication Quarterly* (Graham, 2009; Graham & Herndl, 2013), the *Journal of Medical Humanities* (Graham, 2011), and *Rhetoric Society Quarterly* (Graham & Herndl, 2011). I am very grateful to my reviewers and editors for their diligent commentary and assistance in helping me develop and refine my work in these areas.

Beyond these more formal settings, a great many people have helped significantly by reading drafts, discussing theories, exploring provisional results, and so on. In particular, I'd like to thank Amy Koerber, Bill Keith, Blake Scott, Carla Fehr, Carolyn Miller, Daniel Card, Dave Clark, Diane

Price Herndl, Dorothy Winsor, Greg Wilson, Jenny Watson, John Peppin, Judy Segal, Lee Honeycutt, Leland Poague, Lisa Keränen, Molly Kessler, Patrick Finnerty, and Sheryl Laythem. I am also very grateful for the insightful commentary provided by my reviewers and all the assistance offered by the staff at the University of Chicago Press, among which I am particularly indebted to my editor, David Morrow.

And finally, my never-ending thanks and gratitude to Carl Herndl for being an excellent mentor, collaborator, and friend; to my father not only for raising me but also for introducing me to the broader pain management community; and to Roxi Copland for putting up with me through all of this.

Abbreviations

AAC	Arthritis Advisory Committee
AAPM	American Academy of Pain Management
ACR	American College of Rheumatology
ACR-NEMA	American College of Radiology–National Electrical Manufactures Association
CBD	calibration by detour
CDER	Center for Drug Evaluation and Research
DAC	Drug Advisory Committee
DICOM	Digital Imaging and Communications in Medicine
EBM	evidence-based medicine
FDA	Food and Drug Administration
FMS	fibromyalgia syndrome
IASP	International Association for the Study of Pain
MIC	medical-industrial complex
MPG	Midwest Pain Group (pseudonym)
NFA	National Fibromyalgia Association
PR/WT	principles of rarefication/warranting topoi
RCT	randomized controlled trial

Introduction

At ten feet high and four feet square, artist Mark Collen's *Hey Doc, Have You Figured It Out Yet?* (fig. I.1) suggests a nearly insolvable puzzle. Beyond its impressive size, the work includes a dizzying array of complex medical images including X-rays, sonograms, and CT scans. These images are repeated around the circumference of five different, yet connected cylinders that offer the promise, but not the realization, of alignment. Read against the artist's statement, the "frustration" is palpable, the repetition monotonous. Constructed in a style reminiscent of a "cryptex," this sculpture represents the extreme difficulty confronted both by clinicians who study pain and patients who seek relief. The very idea of a cryptex was invented by Dan Brown for his internationally best-selling *The Da Vinci Code*. An amalgam of cryptology, the study and practice of hiding information, and codex, a bound collection of scrolls (information), a cryptex is a secret store of information that can only be accessed through careful and diligent code breaking. In Brown's narrative, Robert Langdon (professor of symbology and *Da Vinci Code* protagonist) must use all his intellectual acumen to break the cryptex's code and retrieve the hidden information—all while avoiding (and sometimes confronting) a complex array of agendas stemming from secret organizations and powerful institutions.

With this in mind, the cryptex is a remarkably apropos metaphor for the plight of not only the pain patient but also the pain clinician. Pain is a greatly vexing constellation of phenomena for contemporary medicine. In many cases, the causes are unknown; in others, the causes are manifold. Furthermore, treatment options are often a veritable nightmare of multidisciplinary multiplicity. The education and training of physicians tells them that the secrets they seek lie in the code of the human body. In

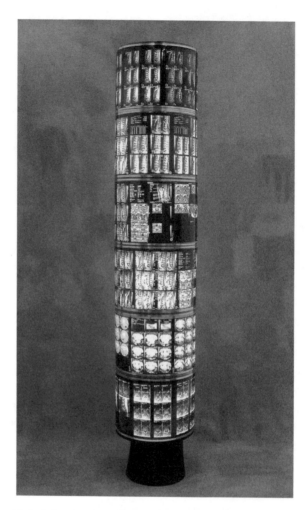

FIGURE I.I. Mark Collen, *Hey Doc, Have You Figured It Out Yet?* According to the artist, "This piece represents the frustration both on the part of the physician and patient in diagnosing and treating chronic pain. It is not unusual for doctors to order the same test over and over again in hopes of understanding the cause of chronic pain. It also exemplifies how the patient often puts the onus on the physician to find the problem and cure it. In reality, it should be a team effort and in many cases there is no cure." (From the Pain Exhibit at painexhibit .org, reprinted with permission.)

medical school, residency, and state-required continuing medical education, they have learned that, eventually, science will prevail. It will crack any code. It will solve any puzzle, if only through continued scrutiny and the agency of ever more sophisticated technologies. Yet at the same time, the question of pain persists. Recognizing this dilemma, clinicians over the past century have published numerous works on pain with suggestive titles like *The Mystery of Pain* (Hinton, 1914), *The Puzzle of Pain* (Melzack, 1973), *The Challenge of Pain* (Melzack & Wall, 1982), and "The Complexity of Pain" (Stevens, 1999). These titles are but a few of the thousands of theoretical treatises, research studies, and clinical trials that have addressed the mysteries of pain. And, certainly, researchers and clinicians studying pain have made great strides throughout medical history. Nevertheless, the cryptex that contains the secrets of pain remains largely unsolved. Clinicians who treat pain routinely grapple with challenging philosophical issues that go to the core of Western science while working in a highly regulated environment. Pain defies modernist categorization.

Indeed, pain's challenge to modernity has been well recognized in social scientific and humanistic studies of health and medicine. Cultural theorist David B. Morris (1991), sociologists Gillian Bendelow and Simon Williams (1995), and historian Roselyn Rey (1993) have each identified a strong tension among various conceptions of pain. Specifically, they note how latent Cartesian dualism underscoring disciplinary paradigms has resulted in individual health-care practitioners who have *either* a physiological *or* a psychological understanding of pain. Morris's work here is especially informative. It is not only representative of the general thrust of the explosion of nonclinical pain scholarship in the early 1990s; it is also widely considered the authoritative work on the topic. Indeed, as of this writing, *The Culture of Pain* boasts over 600 citations indexed on Google Scholar. Morris's book is noteworthy for identifying what he dubs "the myth of two pains":

> Modern culture rests upon an underlying belief so strong that it grips us with the force of a founding myth. Call it the Myth of Two Pains. We live in an era when many people believe—as a basic, unexamined foundation of thought— that pain comes divided into separate types: physical and mental. These two types of pain, so the myth goes, are as different as land and sea. You feel physical pain if your arm breaks, and you feel mental pain if your heart breaks. Between these two different events we seem to imagine a gulf so wide and deep that it might as well be filled by a sea that is impossible to navigate. (p. 9)

Morris's analysis is a thoughtful and thoroughgoing enactment of post-modern cultural criticism. It keenly examines how medical science, clinical practice, and the larger cultural formations that surrounded them in the late 1980s and early 1990s replicate the binaries of modernity, specifically the mind/body dichotomy. And while this was superb scholarship for its time, medicine and cultural studies have both come a long way since 1991.

Contemporary pain medicine is no longer binary; it has become multiple. Research and clinical practice in pain management exists at a nexus of massive multidisciplinarity with treatment options from at least twenty different medical subspecialties ranging from neurology and rheumatology to psychology and physical therapy. Furthermore, pain scientists and physicians had begun to recognize, even before Morris, Bendelow and Williams, and Rey were writing, the pernicious effects of Cartesian dualisms in pain science. Indeed, as psychological researchers John C. Liebeskind and Linda A. Paul note in *Annual Review of Psychology* in 1977:

> While it is often useful to distinguish between various aspects of pain experience [e.g. "sensory-discriminative" versus "motivational-affective" components], other dichotomous terms used in an attempt to specify the origin of pain ("physiological" versus "psychological," "organic" versus "functional") connote a Cartesian dualism and should have been discarded long ago. The use of such terms promotes an unfortunate division of pain patients into those seen to have "real" versus those seen to have "imagined" pain and may lead to inappropriate or insufficient treatment offered to the latter. (p. 42)

Since this time, pain medicine has seen the emergence of a wide variety of groups of clinicians working at local, national, and international levels who are dedicated to a nonbinary, nonreductive approach to solving the pain cryptex. Would-be agentive organizations of pain management clinicians have been striving to change the way practitioners think about and treat pain. I would argue that this coalition of groups is working to foster what Bruno Latour (1991) has famously called a "nonmodern" science—that is, one that rejects and bridges the mind/body duality.[1] Certainly, the most popular term for the new and integrated approach to pain highlights its efforts at nonmodernity: the biopsychosocial model. Indeed, the multiple resonances between the biopsychosocial model and Latourian notions of nonmodernity are so strong that it is worth quoting at length from the opening pages of one of the founding works of biopsychosocial theory, McDaniel, Hepworth, and Doherty's (1992) *Medical Family Therapy*:

Once upon a time, when the problems people brought to a therapist's office could be neatly divided into psychosocial and physical domains, many therapists persuaded themselves that they dealt only with the psychosocial part of life. These therapists did not pursue an understanding of the place of medical illness in the patient's personal and family life because physical health problems were the province of other professionals. Patients with medical problems many have received compassion and support from these therapists but not comprehensive therapy. And few therapists actively collaborated with physicians and other health professionals in the treatment of patients. It is as if patients and families checked their bodies at the door of the therapist's office. The days of innocence are over. *We now know that human life is a seamless cloth spun from biological, psychological, social, and cultural threads; that patients and families come with bodies as well as minds, feelings, interaction patterns, and belief systems; that there are no biological problems without psychosocial implications, and no psychosocial problems without biological implications. Like it or not, therapists are dealing with biological problems, and physicians are dealing with psychosocial problems. The only choice is whether to do integrated treatment well or do it poorly.* (pp. 1–2, emphasis added)

While the biopsychosocial model was something of a flash in the pan for its intended audience of mainstream psychiatrists, it has increasingly become a cornerstone of cross-disciplinary approaches to pain. Advocates of this nonmodern approach have been actively working to transform the multidisciplinary nexus of pain science in accordance with the biopsychosocial model. In establishing this new and nonreductive approach, these practitioners hope to usher in a new era of multidisciplinarity that would result in more effective and holistic treatment for those in pain. Given these changes in the scientific and clinical landscape, a fresh exploration of pain is certainly warranted.

Subsequently, *The Politics of Pain Medicine* chronicles my exploration of various efforts to calibrate the wide variety of disciplinary practices that, when taken as a whole, authorize a biopsychosocial approach to pain. "Calibration" is philosopher Annemarie Mol's (2002) term for efforts to integrate conflicting approaches to medical care. My exploration of multidisciplinary pain medicine will focus on the calibrating efforts at local, disciplinary, and federal levels, exploring along the way the Midwest Pain Group (MPG),[2] the American Academy of Pain Management (AAPM), and the International Association for the Study of Pain (IASP), the disciplines of pathology, radiology, and diagnostics, as well as the Food and Drug Administration (FDA) and their interfaces with and situation within medical disciplines and regulatory bodies. The MPG was a collaborative educational initiative, advocacy effort, and referral network for clinicians from more than twenty different disciplines and subspecialties in a midsize midwestern city. What began as a multidisciplinary journal club evolved quickly into a series of interdependent efforts by more than one hundred members to transform the way pain management was practiced in the region and the state. The AAPM is the premier national organization for multidisciplinary pain management. It offers credentialing, educational, and advocacy efforts nationally in the United States. The IASP is, as the name suggests, the largest and most well-known international organization of multidisciplinary pain specialists. It too provides credentialing, educational, and advocacy services, but on the world stage. Much of the first half *The Politics of Pain Medicine* is focused on the MPG. Yet this exploration necessarily extends beyond the MPG and into the territories of the AAPM, the IASP, medical disciplines, and federal regulatory agencies.

Efforts to calibrate the many forms of scientific and clinical practice needed to authorize a biopsychosocial approach to pain are nothing if not ambitions. In fact, many members of the MPG, AAPM, and the IASP hope that their efforts will help pave the way for a new approach to medicine in general. Indeed, as one interview subject from the MPG argued, "My honest opinion is that we are not going to solve the problem [of pain], or many of the problems in health care, until we get a new model of the mind-body connection. . . . I think somebody's going to put it together. They could be the Freud of the new, of the current, age" (Landau, ethnographic interview).[3] Finding the Freud of the new era and fostering a change of this magnitude will be no easy task. As the subsequent chapters will elucidate, this process is vexed by challenges that (1) lie at the very core of scientific legitimacy, (2) threaten the reimbursement mechanisms of medical subspecialties, and (3) may destabilize the power structures of Western medicine. In establishing a new approach to pain, clinicians, educators, researchers, and regulators must address these difficulties. They must first overcome strong multidisciplinary conflict. Second, they must also foster substantive change in pain theory. And finally, the MPG, the AAPM, and the IASP must refashion the economic and regulatory structures of Western medicine so as to support the new model. Obviously, overcoming disciplinary conflict and fostering revolutionary change are no easy tasks. Neither is establishing socioeconomic and/or regulatory change. Nevertheless, these are the tasks the subjects of my research have embraced, and these are the processes *The Politics of Pain Medicine* explores.

As I suggested briefly above, recent evolutions in the theoretical and methodological approaches of rhetorical and cultural studies of science and medicine also contribute to my argument that now is the ideal time to revisit pain. As the second half of this book's title—*A Rhetorical-Ontological Inquiry*—suggests, this project allies itself with recent developments in rhetoric, technical communication, and science and technology studies (STS) that aim to place the material and the ontological at the center of inquiry. In the same way that pain science and medicine is working to transcend the binaries of modernity, critical scholars of science and medicine are working through new approaches to inquiry. These new approaches recognize that the binaries of modernity were not so much overcome as reified in postmodern inquiry (Latour, 1993; Mol, 2002; Pickering, 2010; Coole & Frost, 2010). Subsequently, *The Politics of Pain Medicine* aims to capitalize on this newfound potential for productive synergy between pain science's biopsychosocial model and rhetoric and STS's turn toward new materialisms. The goal, here, is to be mutually informative. A rhetorical-ontological study of pain will not only help us better understand contemporary practices of pain science and medicine; it will also contribute to the refinement of our own methods and theories. Indeed, I further hope the results of this inquiry will contribute to a better understanding of pain's clinical and regulatory landscape for those who participate in that landscape on a daily basis.

In order to frame my exploration, this introduction must outline my theoretical and methodological approach to the study of pain science: what is a rhetorical-ontological inquiry? While rhetoric of science has a lengthy pedigree with a long focus on effective argumentation strategies in scientific discourse, I use the term "rhetorical-ontological inquiry" as part of an intentional effort to ally my approach much more closely with multidisciplinary STS and its concomitant focus on sociocultural and material aspects of science and technology. Therefore, this book is as much an exploration of how to conduct a rhetorical-ontological study as it is an exploration of pain medicine. The isolated disciplinary conversations of rhetorical studies and STS have, indeed, made strikingly similar arguments and are thus ripe for hybridization. But how to demonstrate that to my readers? For better or worse, there is no other option than to rehearse the various arguments as a part of my analysis. Doing so is an act of calibration that mirrors the calibrations of the pain management communities.

Of course, in so doing, I run the risk of treading through what for some readers might be overly familiar territory. However, what counts as familiar territory for scholars of rhetoric and technical communication may be entirely novel for my readers from STS, and vice versa. Subsequently, I have endeavored to clearly identify the origin and scope of each discussion of the more isolated disciplinary conversations. To the extent that any particular section is overly familiar to you, I invite you to skim or skip over it and proceed to the subsequent analysis.

Rhetoric and STS Need Each Other

Admittedly, this subheading may provoke ire from rhetoricians and STS scholars alike. Yet, as I have suggested above and will further elaborate below, insights from both rhetorical studies and STS are required to adequately explore recent developments in pain science. The establishment of a nonmodern or biopsychosocial approach to pain requires addressing questions of medical science and practice. And here, I mean practice in a way that transcends the postmodern desire to reduce practice to talk, to representation. Scientific practice and clinical performances involve doing things—poking, prodding, cutting, scanning, drugging—things that have real impacts on real patients, things that cannot be so easily (or ethically) reduced to discourse. Certainly, the history of STS inquiry offers a great number of tools that can assist in the investigation of these medical doings. But STS is still not enough. Not only are the doings of clinical practice permeated by talk (discourse), the educational and advocacy efforts of the MPG, AAPM, and the IASP are dominated by acts of representation, including (re-)presentations of clinical practice designed to (re-)present the perspectives of individual clinicians and coalitional organizations. And here, of course, rhetoric has much to offer. While compelling, the demands of the current case may not be enough to convince some of my readers of the value of this cross-disciplinary proposal. So, additionally, I would argue that the internal discussions of each area of inquiry actually demonstrate the need for increased cooperation and conversation between rhetorical studies and STS.

In making this case, I turn first to the benefits that rhetorical studies can offer STS. In 2008, well-known historian of science Peter Galison published an essay in *Isis* titled "Ten Problems in History and Philosophy of Science." Problems one and three articulate Galison's concern that history and philosophy of science would benefit from more sustained and rigorous attention to the contexts and technologies of argumentation. He argues for an increasing focus on issues of intertextuality and strategies of linguistic and visual argumentative practices in the sciences. Specifically, in problem one, "What is context?," Galison suggests that historians and philosophers of science need to develop a more nuanced approach to issues of context, and further that such an approach needs to be built on the fusion of insights from the contextual approaches of each field (history and philosophy) (p. 112). In so doing, Galison argues that philosophers tend to talk about the context of an argument in terms of what rhetoricians would dub "intertextuality"—that is, the relationships among moments of discourse and argument that led up to and are contemporary with the current argument under analysis. In contrast, Galison suggests that historians tend to intentionally ignore discursive contexts in favor of "political, institutional, industrial, or ideological" aspects of the environment (p. 113).

I would argue this is one place where scholars in rhetorical studies have a great deal to contribute to the broader STS community. The notion of context—alongside audience and purpose—is typically identified by rhetoricians as one of the core features of any moment of discourse, and subsequently has been the subject of much scholarly scrutiny. Certainly the notion of "context" means many different things to many different rhetoricians, and the meaning is most typically—but not always—allied with the notion of context that Galison locates with philosophers. However, it is precisely this rich and nuanced tradition of inquiry into context that has the potential to make rhetorical studies so valuable to STS. While problem one may potentially open up the opportunity for more productive conversations among rhetorical studies and STS disciplines, Galison's third problem is a manifestly clear appeal for the expertise of rhetoricians—even if not by name.

In problem three, Galison argues that historians and philosophers of science lack a nuanced understanding of and vocabulary for the "technologies of argumentation":

When the focus is on scientific practices (rather than discipline-specific scientific results per se), what are the concepts, tools, and procedures needed at a given time to construct an acceptable scientific argument? We already have some good examples of steps toward a history and philosophy of practices: instrument making, probability, objectivity, observation, model building, and collecting. We are beginning to know something about the nature of thought experiments—but there is clearly much more to learn. The same could be said for scientific visualization, where, by now, we have a large number of empirical case studies but a relatively impoverished analytic scheme for understanding how visualization practices work. So, cutting across subdisciplines and even disciplines, what is the toolkit of argumentation and demonstration—and what is its historical trajectory? (p. 116)

Here Galison outlines what he sees as an important new research endeavor for historians and philosophers. He does not explicitly invite rhetoricians to join in this conversation. In fact, I am not aware of any moment in Galison's oeuvre where he specifically addresses rhetorical studies as a discipline. Nevertheless, this call for increased research along these lines is the ideal location for an increased intersection between STS and rhetorical studies. Indeed, rhetoricians have a long history (2,500 years, in fact) of exploration into both the contexts and technologies of argumentation. This research tradition—which begins with the pre-Socratics and is exemplified in a long list of thinkers including Aristotle, Cicero, Quintilian, Vico, Nietzsche, Bakhtin, Burke, and a wide variety of contemporary scholars—can offer a ready-made and nuanced approach to the gaps that Galison notes in STS. Furthermore, a great deal of more recent scholarship has been devoted to exploring the technologies of visualization and visual argumentation,[4] and there is a strong history (particularly in the English-rhetoric tradition[5]) of exploring the relationship between scientific investigation and the development of visuals and data displays for a wide variety of different settings. My work here draws on each of these intellectual traditions as a part of my demonstrative suggestion for a combined approach to science and medicine.

Furthermore, Galison is not the only STS scholar who identifies the need for increased engagement with the insights that can be found in rhetorical studies. Philosopher of science and technology Steve Fuller has been interfacing with rhetorical studies since at least 1999. Furthermore, in *The Philosophy of Science and Technology Studies* (2006), Fuller explicitly calls for multidisciplinary engagements with

the debating teams affiliated with the Departments of Speech, Rhetoric, and Communications Studies across college campuses in the United States. Their grassroots initiatives [are] consolidated as the science policy forum convened by the American Association for the Rhetoric of Science and Technology, or AARST. (p. 174)

Fuller's invitation here is grounded in the broad recognition that scientists can no longer maintain the fiction of isolation and political disinterest. With increasing frequency, scientists are being called to participate publicly in the management of divisive political issues. Prominent examples include climate change, H1N1, BSE (mad cow disease), genetic engineering, and nuclear power. Indeed, with such issues, it is considered a matter of course to bring a spate of scientific experts to Washington to provide congressional testimony. As science continues its prominent location within political decision making, attention must be paid to the rhetorical and argumentative dimensions of such debate. And hence, we find another entrée for rhetorical studies into the broader STS conversation. Examples of rhetorical scholarship addressing the role of science in public policy are too numerous to name. A few prominent examples, however, include Lisa Keränen's *Scientific Characters* (2010), Carl Herndl and Stewart Brown's *Green Culture* (1996), Craig Waddell's "The Role of Pathos in the Decision-Making Process" (1990), and Alan Gross's "The Role of Rhetoric in Public Understandings of Science" (1994).

As the introduction to this section suggested, the internal discourse of rhetorical studies also suggests a strong need for increased interface with STS. I begin my exploration with an infamous—among rhetoricians of science, anyway—critique of the discipline offered by Dilip Gaonkar (1997). His "The Idea of Rhetoric in the Rhetoric of Science" was so scathing and subsequently so much discussed that many scholars in the rhetoric of science are, quite frankly, tired of hearing about it. I return to this critique here not so much to revisit the theoretical problems—some of which were quite serious—of early rhetoric of science as to celebrate a new era of scholarship that I believe is finally overcoming the challenges leveled by Gaonkar so long ago. (And in large part, I find this due to the increasing success rhetoricians have found in integrating STS theory into their scholarship.)

The core of Gaonkar's critique involves two key issues: (1) the "thinness" of rhetorical theory and (2) the legacy of humanist agency theory in rhetorical studies. In terms of "thinness," Gaonkar argues that rhetorical theory is overly plastic and adaptable and thus lacks explanatory clarity and precision. His argument stems from the correct assertion that rhetorical studies began (with Aristotle and the Sophists) as a series of generative dictums. Indeed, the earliest works on rhetoric are treaties on the most effective means for generating arguments. They were the textbooks—to use an anachronism—of the day for the aristocracy of ancient Greece who needed to learn the art of civic participation for all manner of political and judicial debates. This legacy provides rhetorical studies with a highly adaptable vocabulary designed to help the progenitors to politicians and lawyers develop effective arguments for whatever situation might arise. These dictums were not originally intended to be used as an analytic frame and have required significant adaptation and refinement to be deployed effectively for scholarly inquiry. In objecting to the thinness of rhetorical theory, Gaonkar contraposes then-recent research in the sociology of scientific knowledge (SSK). Specifically, he argues that "SSK has developed into a complex empirical research program that displays considerable internal variation in theory and methodology, while [rhetoric of science] remains little more than an uncoordinated research initiative carried out by a handful of committed individuals" (p. 42). This is certainly damning criticism, to say the least, but it is also a product of its time—a time that, I would argue, has passed for rhetorical studies of science.

While I agree with Gaonkar that the instrumentalist focus on early texts in rhetorical studies provides a limited range of analytic techniques—that the vocabulary of classical rhetorical theory can be used to describe an argumentative technique (for example, a specific trope or mode of claim building)—the approach sometimes fails to capture issues like the role of larger sociocultural and/or materialist forces that surround and interpenetrate argument. Of course, it should be noted that the two approaches are not mutually exclusive. In fact, prominent STS scholars like Donna Haraway (see, for example, *Modest_Witness*, 2002) artfully deploy the tools of classical rhetoric—for instance, the identification of specific tropes and figures—as a part of their interrogation of ideological issues in the cultures of technoscience. In fact, the fusion of scholarly approaches derived from rhetorical theory and critical/cultural studies has become commonplace in rhetorical studies and is finding increased purchase (with the inclusion of STS) in rhetorics of science and technology. A few especially noteworthy examples come from the work of J. Blake Scott (2003, 2004), Amy Koerber (2006a, 2006b), Carl Herndl (2002), Herndl and Brown (1996), Wilson and Herndl (2007), and so on.

Beyond these intradisciplinary calls for cross-disciplinarity, *The Politics of Pain Medicine* argues that scholars of rhetoric and STS have reached an exciting moment of theoretical symmetry. Scholars from both areas of inquiry have recently embraced and argued for intellectual and scholarly approaches to science, technology, and medicine grounded in what's become known as "new materialisms." And it is this new synergy that constitutes an excellent ground for a more thorough establishment of rhetorical-ontological inquiry as a significant contributor to the broader STS project. The remainder of the theoretical work in this introduction will be devoted to exploring these arguments of new materialisms and reflecting on how the combined efforts of STS scholars and rhetoricians alike can contribute to fleshing out new materialist approaches to science, technology, and medicine.

New Materialisms, STS, and Rhetoric

"New materialisms" is a term used by STS scholars like Diana Coole and Samantha Frost (2010) to describe a growing interest in and emphasis on the material/matériel. Here "material" is inextricably heteroglossic and refers both to the matter of physical reality and the conditions of economic production and social stratification. The introduction to Coole and Frost's *New Materialisms* outlines key issues at stake for STS scholars vis-à-vis new materialisms. Several of these themes also lie at the core of *The Politics of Pain Medicine* and its rhetorical-ontological inquiry. Specifically, these include (1) the recognition of new ontological orientation in STS scholarship, (2) an increased focus on biopolitical and bioethical issues in contemporary technoscience, and (3) a reengagement with the socioeconomic conditions of everyday life (p. 7). And out of these issues arise necessary correlative questions about agency and the extent to which it is circumscribed by both physical and economic determinisms.

Traditional rhetoric of science and SSK/social constructivist approaches in STS have focused—somewhat myopically—on internal scientific discourse to the exclusion of the institutional and the material. Recognizing this issue, many scholars have called for a reincorporation of materiality in rhetoric and STS. Of course, as mentioned above, "materiality" means different things to different people. For some, this call for materiality is a call to investigate the economic and institutional forces that surround discourse (Haraway, 1997, 1998; Herndl, 2002; Kinsella, 2005; Latour, 1993, 1999; Scott, 2003; to name just a few). For others, however, the argument for materiality focuses on the objects of reality and might more aptly be described as an argument for a reincorporation of ontology (Bennett, 2010a, 2010b; Jack, 2010; Mol, 1999, 2002; Pickering, 2010; Graham, 2009; Harman, 2009; Herndl, 2002; Lynch, 2009; Marback, 2008; Rickert, 2013). Regardless of the focus (matter or money), these demands for a return to ontology and materiality in rhetorical studies and STS are gaining volume and momentum. As Coole and Frost note, "Everywhere we look, it seems to us, we are witnessing scattered but insistent demands for more materialist modes of analysis and for new ways of thinking about matter and processes of materialization" (p. 2). As suggested above, the arguments of new materialisms can be enacted with a variety of different overlapping foci—but these are foci of the same arguments made by the same scholars. There is no physical-material camp and no socioeconomic-material camp. When it comes to new materialisms, it's a both/and rather than an either/or approach.

Scholars that focus on the physical tend to focus on the role of matter—the brute objects composed of colliding particles—in the laboratory and experimental practices. In STS, this mode of new materialism is enacted under a wide variety of different theoretical rubrics. A few prominent examples include Hans-Jörg Rheinberger's (2010) epistemology of the concrete, Graham Harman's (2009) object-oriented metaphysics, Levi Bryant's (2011) object-oriented ontologies, Jane Bennett's (2010b) vibrant materialism, Andrew Pickering's (2010) nonmodern ontologies, Ian Bogost's (2012) alien phenomenology, and Annemarie Mol's (2002) multiple ontologies. While the theoretical nuances of each these approaches can vary significantly, they each share a strong focus on and engagement with physical objects as one primary locus of analysis. The cases addressed vary widely and include Rheinberger's analysis of model organisms in the biological sciences, Bennett's engagement with a collection of junk in a storm drain, Pickering's interest in robotic turtles, Bogost's study of computer code, Bryant's interrogation of cats and coffee mugs, and Mol's investigation of the clot-matter found in leg veins.

And this newfound focus on the physical-material is not limited to STS. Indeed, many in rhetorical studies now argue, like Marback, that the field's traditional focus on hermeneutics and representation creates a situation wherein "rhetorical studies . . . fails to give the object its due" (p. 53). Even more specifically for the rhetoric of science, Herndl argues that rhetoric needs to embrace "a [new] model of science and scientific argument that integrates the social and the material with the discursive, but which does not abandon the real" (2002, p. 217). Additionally, Lynch argues that rhetoricians of science tend to be blinded to objects through their own particular terministic screens that "deflect attention from material practice" (p. 442). Furthermore, he suggests that "separating the material in the rhetorical prevents rhetorical critics from considering the interanimation of the two and, more specifically, how the relationship with specific material elements influences rhetorical practice" (p. 442). Thankfully, this trend toward anti-material deflection seems to be reversing. The work of a variety of rhetorical scholars is now beginning to address the role of physical objects within a broader material-semiotic milieu. The work of scholars like J. Blake Scott (2003), Jessica J. Mudry (2009), Joanna Ploeger (2009), Elizabeth Parthenia Shea (2008), Rickert (2013), in addition to my own work (Graham, 2009, 2011; Graham & Herndl, 2013; Teston, Graham, Baldwinson, Li & Swift, 2014), has moved strongly in the direction of new materialisms and their object-oriented foci. Indeed, this spate of scholarship interrogates a variety of objects including human blood, genes, particle accelerators, food calories, and pathological conditions alongside inquiry into the rhetorical and discursive issues at work in concert with these objects.

Arguments for a focus on the institutional-material aspects of science have a long pedigree in STS. Indeed, scholars like Donna Haraway, Evelyn Fox Keller, Andrew Pickering, and Bruno Latour are famous across disciplinary boundaries for their work in this area. The most recent work in this line—that is, the scholarship that explicitly identifies itself as new materialist—is intensely revisiting notions of agency, individualism, subjectivity, freedom, and biopolitics within the economic-materialist milieu. For example, Elizabeth Grosz (2010) argues that these issues have typically been addressed—especially in feminist scholarship—through "the discourses of political philosophy, and the debates between liberalism, historical materialism, and postmodernisms regarding the sovereignty and rights of subjects and social groups" (p. 140). Her aim, in contrast, is to reinterpret such notions within an ontological/new materialist idiom. That is, she asks questions about the very nature of freedom within something like an Althusserian (1971) concept of constraint borne of state apparatuses—repressive and ideological. Similarly, Rosi Braidotti (2010) seeks to relocate discussions of embodiment and embodied materialism away from the typical focus on the physical material of biomatter—bones, sinew, lipoproteins, and pathological conditions. Indeed, this argument compellingly suggests that the reinterpretation of embodiment within the economic-material milieu has a great deal to contribute to Foucauldian notions of biopower. Certainly there are myriad number of different research questions which could be (and are being) addressed under the economic material rubric of new materialisms. See Braidotti (2010), Coole (2007), Chow (2010), Grosz (1994), and Rose (2001) for some additional prominent examples. In each of these cases, readers will find the same strong emphasis on reimagining issues of agency, subjectivity, and biopolitics in the light of new materialisms.

Arguments for an institutional-material rhetoric of science typically focus on large scientific institutions and the complicated socioeconomic mechanisms that surround them. Scholars from this camp typically draw on resources from critical/cultural studies and seek to criticize the leveraging of power in material-semiotic networks such as the military and medical industrial complexes. As William Kinsella notes, "Contemporary science and technology are characterized by unprecedented degrees of institutionalization, and that in these settings the locus of agency has shifted increasingly from the individual to large systems of power/knowledge" (2005, p. 303). Interrogating these systems of power/knowledge requires new theoretical and methodological tools—tools that account for institutional-materiality. Recognizing this, Scott (2003) argues for a hybrid rhetorical-cultural study of science wherein the goal "is to map the connections and power relations among science's heterogeneous actors" (p. 355). Reflecting on the affordances of this approach, Scott argues that

> it also departs from the traditional subordination of these notions to the individual text. Rather than accounting for cultural entanglements as a way to situate and elucidate texts, a rhetorical-cultural mapping discusses specific texts as a way to elucidate cultural entanglements. In such an approach, the shifting intertext itself becomes the primary object of study. (p. 355)

In a move that anticipates Galison's interest in context, Scott articulates a way of folding the notion of discursive intertextuality into the more historical-cultural notions of context qua socioeconomic. It is arguments like these that pave the way for highly productive synergies between rhetoric and STS.

Diagnostic Consensus: The Two-World Problem

With this bewildering array of alien phenomenologies, epistemologies of the concrete, institutional-material rhetorics, object-oriented ontologies, vibrant materialities, and biopolitical theories, it can sometimes be hard to see new materialisms as a coordinated endeavor. The plethora of proposed solutions elides the near-complete uniformity of diagnostic consensus. That is, scholars from fields as far ranging as rhetoric, philosophy, sociology, political science, and history have all come to agree on the central failing in Western intellectual history, the so-called two-world problem (see fig. I.2): the series of bifurcations that includes the subject/object, culture/nature, and mind/body dichotomies. These binaries not only establish the core territory of modernism, they create an epistemological crisis. This crisis is what Harman (2011) refers to as "the problem of access" and Bryant (2011) as "the epistemic fallacy." The irreversible, unbridgeable dichotomy between the subject and the object forces a constant reengagement with the question of whether or not the subject has access to the object. Elaborating Latour's critique of modernist epistemology, Bryant argues:

> As a consequence of the two world schema, the question of the object, of what substances are, is subtly transformed into the question of how and whether we know objects. The question of objects becomes the question of a particular relationship between humans and objects. This, in turn, becomes questions of whether or not our representations map onto reality. (p. 16)

Of course, at the outset, there doesn't appear to be all that much "new" about new materialisms. The rejection of modernist and/or Cartesian binaries has a long pedigree in postmodern thought tracing back to the (proto-)postmodernist Martin Heidegger and his hermeneutic circle and popping up in a wide variety of scholarship ranging from Derrida's deconstruction of the metaphysics of presence to Rorty's critique of the mirror of nature.

Indeed, the rejection of modernist binaries has similarly been a staple of STS for decades, finding perhaps its fullest expression in Haraway's *Simians, Cyborgs, and Women* (1991) where she recognizes the incredible pervasiveness of the two-world problem (although not by that name) and the litany of dualisms it authorizes:

> To recapitulate, certain dualisms have been persistent in Western traditions; they have all been systemic to the logics and practices of domination of women, of people of colour, nature, workers, animals—in short, domination of all constituted others, whose task is to mirror the self. Chief among these troubling dualisms are self/other, mind/body, culture/nature, male/female, civilized/primitive, reality/appearance, whole/part, agent/resource, maker/made, active/passive, right/wrong, truth/illusion, total/partial, God/man. (p. 177)

So if the recognition of this proliferation of dualisms is such well-trodden territory, one might be justifiably compelled to ask what makes new materialisms *new*. Why do I point to it as an appropriate path forward if it appears repetitive in its founding diagnosis?

The newness of new materialisms comes from its full acceptance of Latour's well-known critique of postmodernism—namely, that despite claims to the contrary, postmodernism's rejection of positivism/modernism does not so much deconstruct the two-world problem as it does reify it. As he notes, "Postmodernism is a symptom, not a fresh solution. It lives under the modern Constitution, but no longer believes in the guarantees the Constitution offers" (1993, p. 46). Translating from Latourian, this is the argument that the postmodernists do not actually reject the two-world hypothesis. They instead reify it, privileging the "other" side, placing subject over object, words over things, culture over nature.

Indeed, Annemarie Mol highlights the pervasiveness of this postmodern reversal in her objection to the now standardized disease/illness distinction in humanistic and social scientific studies of health and medicine. In a passage that has striking parallels with Liebeskind and Paul's criticism of pain science, Mol (2002) argues:

> Social scientists have made it their trade to listen for feelings when they interview patients. And they have persistently and severely criticized doctors for neglecting psychosocial matters, for being ever so concerned about keeping wounds clean while they hardly ever ask their patients what being wounded means to them. In addition to attending to blood sugar levels, bad arteries, wounds, and other physicalities, or so social scientists have been arguing in all kinds of ways, physicians should attend to what patients experience. This is how they have come to phrase it: in addition to *disease*, the object of biomedicine, something else is of importance too, a patient's *illness*. Illness here stands for a patient's interpretations of his or her disease, the feelings that accompany it, the life events it turns into. (p. 9)

Here we see the typical postmodern intellectual move in action: a rejection of modernism's hegemonic focus on the so-called real replaced with a new discursive hegemony where the real is elided entirely. Or as Mol puts it, "In a world of meaning, nobody is in touch with the reality of diseases, everybody 'merely' interprets them. There are different interpretations around, and 'the disease'—forever unknown—is nowhere to be found. The disease *recedes* behind the interpretations" (pp. 11–12). (I use the word "hegemony" very consciously here.)

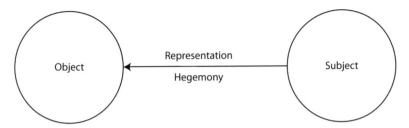

FIGURE I.2. The two-world of modernity and postmodernity. Both modernist and postmodernist metaphysics offer a bifurcated world that separates subjects from objects. Where modernism construes the relationship between subject and object as one of representation (proposed correspondence), postmodernism offers a theory of hegemonic relationality.

Bryant echoes the insights of both Mol and Latour and, in so doing, identifies a second predominant fallacy of Western thought—"the hegemonic fallacy" (p. 131). The hegemonic fallacy, which also arises from the two-world problem, is predicated on the postmodern reversal of the two-world binaries. That is, where modernism privileges the real object over the perceiving subject, postmodernism recasts the object as an extension of the subject's perception, and the object becomes an epiphenomenon of the subject (the death of the referent). For Bryant, it is this totalizing subject that gives rise to hegemony critiques and is equally, again, of the two-world problem. As readers of *Reassembling the Social* (2005) will recognize, Bryant's rejection of the hegemonic fallacy also echoes Latour's concern that actor-network theory (ANT) is too often "confused with a postmodern emphasis on the critique of the 'Great narratives' and 'Eurocentric' or 'hegemonic' standpoint" (2005, p. 11). Indeed, much like Bryant, Latour caustically dismisses scholarship on hegemonic forces as accounts of an "invisible agency" (p. 53). As he declares, "In ANT, it is not permitted to say, 'No one mentions it. I have no proof but I know there is some hidden actor at work behind the scene.' This is conspiracy theory, not social theory" (p. 53). And while I'm not willing to go as far as Latour in rejecting the role of elided forces, as I will explore in chapter 6, the too-easy deployment of hegemonic narratives obscures viable possibilities for positive change in pain science and pharmaceutical regulation.

Ultimately, the two-world problem and its twin fallacies (epistemic and hegemonic) help to explain both the unity and the dizzying array of new materialisms. To transcend the two-world problem is to transcend both the epistemic and hegemonic fallacies simultaneously. This, of course, presents any work attempting to do so with a previously inconceivable task. For the two-world problem authorizes the traditional divisions between research projects in rhetoric of science and STS. That is, investigations of laboratory practice and science-policy debates are required to be distinctly different tasks under the two-world problem. In contrast, a thoroughgoing embrace of new materialisms and its attendant rejection of the epistemic and hegemonic fallacies requires a dissolution of not only the modernist binaries but also the boundaries typically enforced between complementary areas of scholarship. As Latour (1999) puts it:

> There is thus no longer much sense in pursuing in isolation questions like "How can a mind know the world outside?" "How can the public participate in technical expertise" "How can we protect nature from human greed?" "How can we build a livable political order?" Very quickly inquiries into these matters stumble over so many aporias, since the definitions of nature, society, morality and the Body Politic were all produced together, in order to create the most powerful and most paradoxical of all powers: a politics that does away with politics, the inhumane laws of nature that keep humanity from falling into inhumanity. (p. 293)

Separating these questions from one another in this book would be doubly inappropriate given the primary subject under investigation. As I have alluded to above, the pursuit of a biopsychosocial, nonmodern theory of pain is borne of a nearly identical diagnosis of the failure of the two-world problem. Indeed, the two-world problem, in its various instantiations, and through its various fallacious corollaries, simultaneously *gives rise to and authorizes* the primary problems in pain medicine (the myth of two pains, the rejection of subjective patient report) as well as many of the central theoretical problems in rhetoric of science and STS (the death of agency, the illness/disease dichotomy, the incommensurability thesis, the problem of expertise). See figure I.3 for a more detailed schematic.

Subsequently, it is an essential aim of *The Politics of Pain Medicine* to investigate and explore what it means to simultaneously overcome the two-world problem in rhetorical studies, STS, and pain medicine. Additionally, figure I.3 serves as a relational map in two ways. Most obviously, it (1) maps the various theoretical, practical, and ethical problems that arise from the two-world hypothesis and (2) details the potential for productive synergies among new materialist rhetorical studies, nonmodern STS, and a biopsychosocial approach to pain medicine. In recognizing this, I hope all three areas may be improved through this colocated exploration. And lest there be any doubt on the possible reciprocal contributions rhetorical-ontological inquiry and biopsychosocial pain management can

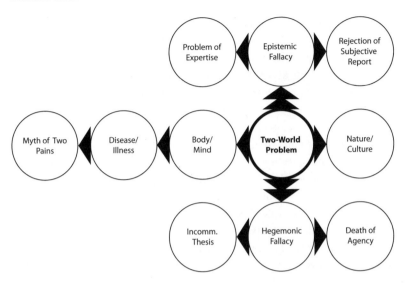

FIGURE I.3. The two-world problem in pain, rhetoric, and STS. This schematic details how the two-world problem, as the central conceit in (post-)modernist thought, simultaneously gives rise to and authorizes the major problems of both pain science and rhetorical-STS inquiry. The two-world hypothesis creates the epistemic fallacy, which gives rise to the problem of expertise in rhetoric/STS and the rejection of subjective patient report in pain medicine. The two-world problem further creates the hegemonic fallacy and, in so doing, the incommensurability thesis and the death of agency become necessary corollaries. And finally, the two-world problem also legitimizes the manifold dualisms (nature/culture, body/mind, disease/illness, myth of two pains) recognized by contemporary medical science and postmodern rhetoric and STS.

make to each another, allow me to highlight one of my interview subject's deft criticism of the original (post-)modern two-world situation of this project:

> You used in your introduction to this study the idea of epistemology and hermeneutics. I don't know how you're going to use those words. There's been 2,500 years of philosophical polemic that there's an ontological difference [between epistemology and hermeneutics], but there's not at a neurophysiological level. Internal versus external, that is, the subjectivity of consciousness. . . . To separate epistemology and hermeneutics is contextual only. At the neurobiological level they are the same. (Michelson, interview)

Here, Dr. Michelson, an orthopedist, rejects any dualist separation between knowledge and meaning and does so simultaneously for both philosophical and neurobiological reasons. As will be seen in the chapters that follow, this kind of detour through philosophy becomes somewhat commonplace as part of efforts to found a biopsychosocial pain. And as the clinicians involved in my inquiry reject not only medical disciplinary boundaries but also the traditional divisions among the humanities, arts, and sciences, a great deal can be learned for rhetorical-ontological inquiry.

Finally, figure I.3 also provides something of a road map for the work of *The Politics of Pain Medicine*. It helps to identify the central foundation from which the spiraling corollaries of the two-world problem emerge. Figure I.3 identifies the central origin of what might, through the lens of traditional scholarly boundaries, seem a collection of somewhat disparate chapters. Chapter 1 explores an intermingling between the history of pain and the incommensurability thesis. Chapters 2 and 3 focus on the relationship between physical materiality and the rhetorical as the MPG attempts to find its own version of biopsychosocial pain. Chapters 4, 5, and 6 offer an exploration of ontological adjudication in institutional spaces, at one point detouring through the history of neuroimaging and in other places exploring disciplinary and institutional disagreements over the ontologies of fibromyalgia syndrome and the sinus headache. At the root of all these endeavors is the attempt to transcend the two-world problem and in so doing develop a robust rhetorical-ontological account of pain science and medicine. A major part of that effort will be, as mentioned above, to document and investigate the modes of calibration that bring together researchers and practitioners who subscribe to different approaches to pain. In so doing, *The Politics of Pain Medicine* will offer a taxonomy of calibrating practices used by the multidisciplinary pain medicine practitioners, researchers, and advocates. The ultimate taxonomy will include a range of modes of calibration (cross-ontological calibration, constitutive calibration, rarefactive calibration, calibration by detour), authorizing institutional resources (principles of rarefaction, institutions of rarefaction, black-box technologies), and discursive instantiations (stasis debate, warranting topoi, trope shifting). I leave the details this taxonomy to chapters 2–6, which follow chapter 1's historical investigation of the emergence of the many pain practices that require calibration.

An Ontological History of Pain

O Death the Healer, scorn thou not, I pray, To come to me: of cureless ills thou art The one physician. Pain lays not its touch Upon a corpse. —Aeschylus

I would say that pain is part of the glory, or the tremendous mystery of life. And that if anything, it's a kind of privilege to stand so close to such an incredible miracle. —Simone Taylor (Klassen, 2001, p. 193)

Whether it is Aeschylus's horrible pain that can only be alleviated by death, Simone Taylor's description of the glorious pain of childbirth, or a garden-variety headache, pain is a nearly ubiquitous to the human condition. Nevertheless, I imagine most people would be hardpressed to come up with a succinct definition of "pain." Pain defies categorization. The multiplicity of pain is probably best encapsulated in the title of one of the premier French medical journals for the study of pain, *Douleurs* (Pains). By adding an *s* to the more common mass noun *douleur*, French physicians and researchers are highlighting pain's multiplicity. Indeed, it is quite tempting to follow the lead of French pain clinicians and adopt "pains" rather than "pain" in this work. However, I have largely declined to do so for two reasons: It is not a linguistic move that biopsychosocial Anglophone pain researchers are making, and "pains" simply has too long a history in nonmedical Anglophone contexts (for example, in idioms like "to take great pains").

Linguistics aside, there are myriad physical, emotional, social, and cultural causes of pain and an equally myriad number of physical and emotional symptoms and manifestations. Pain management, if attempted, is often only a temporary process of symptom suppression—something done to help one cope as the underlying mechanism of illness or injury is addressed. Of course, this is not always the case. Seldom does one think of "curing" a headache. You take your preferred painkiller and wait for it to pass, all headaches forgotten until the next one. However, pain management may be different still in the case of pain as part of chronic depression. In this case there is a cause: the depression. But is there a cause of the cause? Is the depression the result of a traumatic experience, a neurotransmitter imbalance, or both, or neither? Will the pain subside with the treatment of the depression? Pain as a phenomenon and pain management as a practice are truly problematic. The complexities of each are inextricably tied up with each other and with the illness at hand—if there is one.

Of course, it's not only rhetoricians, STS scholars, and cultural theorists who have trouble formulating or articulating a succinct understanding of pain. The many natures of pain and the appropriate practices for pain management are topics of vigorous debate in and among many health-care disciplines. Pain management is an area of practice and a certifiable subspecialty in many disciplines and subspecialties—including but not limited to anesthetic medicine, neurology, psychology, pharmacy, physical therapy, and nursing. However, no two of these disciplines conceive of pain or practice pain management in quite the same way. This issue is recognized by multidisciplinary coalitional groups such as the International Association for the Study of Pain (IASP). The IASP developed the first internationally recognized definition of pain at the Fourth World Congress on Pain in 1984, and it has continued to be revised by the IASP Task Force on Taxonomy. This official IASP definition explicitly attempts to "represent agreement between diverse specialties including anesthesiology, dentistry, neurology, neurosurgery, neurophysiology, psychiatry, and psychology."[1]

Despite the laudable nature of scientific and humanist work aimed at overcoming the myth of two pains, when viewed through the lens of the two-world hypothesis (as is typically the case) only a small portion of the conflicting issues present in pain management are manifest. In fact, the historiography of pain is typically troubled twice-over by the two-world hypothesis. In the first instance, humanist and social scientific historians tend to read pain through the disease/illness dichotomy and thus present the well-trodden argument that overly biomechanical pain scientists ignore the subjective and affective dimensions of pain as illness (Morris, 1991; Bendelow & Williams, 1995; Rey, 1993, 1995; Liebeskind & Paul, 1997). In the second case, humanist and social scientific historians of pain also tacitly deploy the hegemonic fallacy, in that they recount the history of pain science as a successive parade of totalizing paradigms, where theorists and practitioners are locked in the theoretical zeitgeist of the day only to be entirely replaced in their old age by the next generation of scientists who inhabit a new and different world of pain (Melzack, 1973; Melzack & Wall, 1982; Rey, 1993). However, neither of these two-world approaches to the historiography are quite appropriate to the multiplicity of pain, scientific and clinical, historical and contemporary.

Individual pain scientists and clinicians, throughout history, have confronted myriad pains. "Individual" is an essential modifier in that last sentence. It is far too easy to read it as another expression of totalizing theory succession. When I say that pain scientists and clinicians confront myriad pains, I very much do not mean that each successive generation confronted new theories of pain. I mean that Galen, Dr. Leriche, and Dr. Melzack each confronted multiple pains simultaneously in their clinical practices of the second century, 1935, and 1970, respectively. To be sure, each clinician confronted a different (but partially overlapping) set of pains. These simultaneously extant pains fall on either side of and sometimes across the Cartesian divide and have been represented across a variety of medical and scientific disciplines. Here again, it would be too easy to read that last sentence as suggesting that each discipline has its own pain. But as this chapter will demonstrate, that neither was nor currently is the case. Most disciplines exhibit multiple simultaneous pains. Thus, the primary aim of this chapter is to offer an alternative history of pain, one that accounts for the multiplicity of simultaneous extant pains in a new materialist idiom. In so doing, I contribute to new materialist efforts to overcome the two-world problem in humanistic scholarship. Furthermore, this history will also provide essential contextualization for my discussion of the way that these many pains circulate in the contemporary practices of pain management (chapters 2–3), efforts to found and authorize new pain ontologies (chapters 3–4), and the networks of disciplines and regulatory agencies that surround those efforts (chapters 5–6).

Macrohistory without Incommensurability

Historiographers have, from time to time, offered a distinction of scope in regard to their work: macrohistory versus microhistory. While there is no easy and agreed-upon line of demarcation to be drawn between these two historiographic scopes, the difference is easy to see on the margins. A macrohistory of evolutionary science, for example, might trace the sweeping changes from Lamarck and Lyell through Darwin and Huxley and on to the modern synthesis.[2] In contrast, a microhistory could offer a detailed analysis of the historical contexts that contributed to Charles Darwin and Alfred Russel Wallace's virtually simultaneous development of the theory of evolution by natural selection. In the first case, the historiographic scope is a span of more than a hundred years. In the second case, the focus may fall on a single decade or less. In contemporary history of science and technology, microhistory is now the dominant form of inquiry. Ironically ushered in by the most macro of macrohistorians, Thomas Kuhn, the shift to social constructivism required an attendant shift in inquiry away from documentation of successive ideas over broad timelines (macrohistory) toward a much more detailed focus on the socio-contextual milieu in which individual ideas incubated (microhistory).

The predominant focus on microhistories over the past several decades means little attention has been paid to updating the practice of macrohistory to account for contemporary and emerging approaches like new materialisms. As such, there remain essentially two primary options for macrohistory of science and technology: the appropriately much-maligned Whig history and the rather more popular (post-)Kuhnian theory succession. *Whig history* was coined by Herbert Butterfield in 1944 to refer to efforts by the Whig Party of England to rewrite English history into a teleological narrative culminating in Whig ascendency. Whig approaches to the history of science and technology remain quite prevalent, especially in histories written by practicing scientists. Whig histories of science present theories currently in vogue as unassailably correct and rewrite the history of science into a teleological narrative that ends in the final and true discovery of the current concepts. Both the Whig approach and the Kuhnian approach are common in contemporary histories of pain, whether those histories were penned by biomedical researchers or more humanistic historians. The Whig approach to pain is, however, particularly common among biomedical researches who craft a narrative that leads eventually toward the current scientific theory. Fishman and Berger's (2000) *The War on Pain* exemplifies this tradition when identifying the work of René Descartes as essentially accurate:

> Considering that Descartes' methods of exploration were limited to crude microscopes and dissected cadavers, his concept of the sensory nervous system was wonderfully advanced. Pain *does* travel along pathways of nervous,

although not along a single primary interstate, so to speak, but via two main routes.... (p. 9)

Similarly, historian Roselyne Rey (1994) identifies C. S. Sherrington as the first person to develop a "modern theory of pain," indicating that it is somehow more scientifically accurate than its predecessors. Of course, I reject teleological historiography for obvious reasons and also find theory succession to be an inadequate explanatory heuristic given its correlative suggestion that prior theories were discarded in favor of new ones.

More compelling but still ultimately problematic histories of pain are offered in the theory succession tradition. In *The Culture of Pain* (1991), David Morris explicitly references the work of Kuhn in his explanation of the discovery of tic douloureaux/trigeminal neuralgia as a departure from normal puzzle-solving science (pp. 164–165). Perhaps more interesting, however, is the case of world-renowned pain theorist Ronald Melzack, who explicitly and intentionally presents a narrative of theory succession in his canonical *The Puzzle of Pain* (1973) as a way of warranting his "revolutionary" new theory of pain:

> However, when all the theories—from specificity theory onward—are examined together, it is apparent that each successive theory makes an important contribution. Each provides an additional mechanism to explain some of the complex clinical syndromes of experimental data that were previously inexplicable. Despite the seemingly small differences, each change contains a major conceptual idea that has had a powerful impact on research and therapy. (p. 152)

Lest there be any doubt of Melzack's own view of his new theory as a noncumulative developmental episode à la Kuhn, he (with Wall) later writes in *The Challenge of Pain*, the 1982 update to his 1973 classic, "We consider ourselves extremely privileged to have taken part in a genuine scientific revolution in the past two decades" (p. viii). Ultimately, as I argue above, neither the teleological Whig history nor theory succession are appropriate to the manifest multiplicity of pain. The history of pain medicine is a history of multiple practical and theoretical emergences. However, only periodically did a newly emerged theory supplant a prior theory, as the theory succession model would have it. Furthermore, the Kuhnian approach to historiography puts us firmly on the path to social construction, incommensurability theory, and the hegemonic fallacy, all things I hope to avoid. Thus a new approach to macrohistory is required—one that is consonant with the dictates of new materialism.

Now, incommensurability studies, which arise from theory succession historiography, have a long pedigree in history of science and rhetorical studies. Nevertheless, I must reject both Kuhnian historiography and incommensurability theory as both inappropriate to a macrohistory of pain and untenable under the rubric of new materialisms. In short, as I've argued elsewhere (Graham & Herndl, 2013), incommensurability theory is a legacy of the two-world problem. It invokes that problem in at least two ways: Incommensurability is inextricably modernist in that it posits a binary reality composed of a world and a view, and it commits the hegemonic fallacy by offering a totalizing theory of paradigmatic ideology. Mol's multiple-ontologies approach transcends each of these problems by providing a compelling alternative to incommensurability, one that neither is modernist nor commits the hegemonic fallacy. As Mol repeatedly reminds us, postmodern theories of paradigms or ideology are irrevocably perspectival. They are shot through with visual metaphors that serve to (re-)establish the profound modernist separation between a subject and an object, culture and nature, a view and the world.

Indeed, ocular metaphors are pervasive in Kuhn's *Structure of Scientific Revolutions* (1996) and persist through rhetorical inquiry into incommensurability. For example, Kuhn's perspectivalism finds its clearest expression in the title of the tenth chapter in *Structure*: "Revolutions as Changes of World View" (p. 111). In this chapter, as in the others before and after it, Kuhn makes recurrent references to how scientists *see* the world as a result of their paradigms. The gestalt switch metaphor—though troubling for Kuhn—is recurrent. And there is, furthermore, example after example of revolutionary scientists who *see* and inhabit an entirely new world post-paradigm revolution: "The very ease and rapidity with which astronomers saw new things when looking at old objects with old instruments may make us wish to say that, after Copernicus, astronomers lived in a different world. In any case, their research responded as though that were the case" (p. 117). Kuhnian paradigms are fundamentally the goggles through which one sees the world:

> In their most usual form, of course, gestalt experiments illustrate only the nature of the perceptual transformations. They tell us nothing about the role of paradigms or of previously assimilated experience in the process of perception. But on that point there is a rich body of psychological literature, much of it

stemming from the pioneering work of the Hanover Institute. An experimental subject who puts on goggles fitted with inverting lenses initially sees the entire world upside down. At the start his perceptual apparatus functions as it had been trained to function in the absence of goggles, and the result is extreme disorientation, an acute personal crisis. But after the subject has begun to learn to deal with his new world, his entire visual field flips over, usually after an intervening period in which visual is simply confused. Thereafter, objects are again seen as they had been before the goggles were put on. The assimilation of previously anomalous visual field has reacted upon and changed the field itself. Literately as well as metaphorically, the man accustomed to inverting lenses has undergone a revolution transformation of vision. (p. 112)

Even though Kuhn's approach is primarily designed to allow us to escape the never-ending epistemological debates of positivism, falsification, and all the rest, it ultimately recapitulates the two-world problem, committing the epistemic fallacy and dooms us to another four decades (and counting) of fraught and fruitless epistemological debates. In so doing, it also authorizes incommensurability theory's commission of the hegemonic fallacy.

As Kuhn argues time and time again, "The decision to reject one paradigm is always simultaneously the decision to accept another, and the judgment leading to that decision involves the comparison of both paradigms with nature and with each other" (p. 77). Paradigms are totalizing ideological blinders (perspectival metaphor again). They are goggles locked in place that nearly irrevocably impact how one sees the world. Paradigms are so powerful that, according to Kuhn's reading of Max Planck's autobiography, one is more likely to die than change (p. 151): "Proponents of competing paradigms practice their trades in different worlds" (p. 150). Here is the origin of incommensurability and the incommensurability thesis that I reference in the introduction. If members of competing paradigms live in different worlds, then they are fundamentally incapable of communication. This is what Randy Allen Harris refers to as "cosmic incommensurability" or the "situation in which communication is severely hindered because of different perceptions of the 'same' phenomenon, where parties can't communicate coherently because they 'live in different worlds'" (2005, p. 22).

The incommensurability thesis is pervasive in rhetorical studies of cross-disciplinary conflict. It is perhaps most famously exemplified in Herndl, Fennel, and Miller's (1991) canonical analysis of NASA deliberations over whether or not to launch the last space shuttle *Challenger* mission in light of the troubling O-ring data. Ultimately, Herndl, Fennel, and Miller conclude, "Our analysis suggests that the common view that managers at Morton Thiokol were just acquiescing to pressure from NASA is too simple. Rather, it may be that engineers and managers were *unable*, more than unwilling, to recognize data which deviated from that characteristic of their organizational roles" (pp. 302–303, emphasis added). In other words, communication between NASA managers and engineers was incommensurable. They simply lived in different worlds. This passage was, of course, highlighted in Walzer and Gross's (1994) famous objection to the incommensurability analysis in the *Challenger* case. While Walzer and Gross's article ultimately argues for a much more modernist vision of knowledge than I'm willing to endorse, they present compelling data that indicate, in fact, at least some of the NASA managers were able to appreciate the engineer's point of view and changed their minds accordingly. This suggests, in contrast to Herndl, Fennell, and Miller's argument, that those managers who did not appreciate the engineering point of view may well have been more unwilling than unable.

And, this is, of course, but one example among many. Scientists routinely communicate effectively across disciplinary boundaries. Indeed, successful cross-disciplinary collaborations among scientists are well documented in both rhetorical and STS literature. See Star and Griesemer (1989), Galison (2008), Wilson and Herndl (2007), and Bazerman and De Los Santos (2005) for but a few of the most well-known examples in each discipline. Indeed, the manifest ability of scientists to communicate successfully and productively across seemingly incommensurable boundaries has provoked a model of inquiry that looks strikingly like a Kuhnian paradigm crisis for rhetorical studies and STS. When empirical data demonstrates that scientists regularly violate the incommensurability thesis, the thesis is not falsified. Rather, rhetorical and STS analysts invent ad hoc modifications for incommensurability theory in order to explain the current case. Thus we have a proliferation of socio-rhetorical constructs that authorize our analyses of cross-disciplinary communication such as boundary objects (Star & Griesemer), trading zones (Galison), integrative exigencies (Wilson & Herndl), and so on. These socio-rhetorical constructs posit that in cases of successful cross-disciplinary collaboration, there must be something special and extra that authorizes that success. Prominent examples include shared objects of study, spaces of work, sources of funding, or pressing emergencies, any of which might allow certain local cross-disciplinary groups to overcome the incommensurability thesis. Additionally, we also have further modifications such as Harris's incommensurability suite, which posits a series of decreasingly powerful forms of incommensurability, each with weaker predictions of cross-disciplinary conflict.

So, ultimately, and very self-consciously in regard to the irony, I recommend that we (as many have already done) discard the incommensurability paradigm and shift to new materialism and specifically multiple-ontologies theory. In so doing, we have a compelling opportunity to overcome the limits of incommensurability's legacy of modernism and its commission of both the epistemic and hegemonic fallacies. Indeed, where incommensurability describes epistemological differences based on different paradigms that provide competing "perspectives" on a stable reality, the theory of multiple ontologies, in contrast, describes differently situated material activities that produce different objects. One is a theory of seeing and knowing: What you see or know is determined by the theoretical position or paradigm from which you look. The other is a theory of doing and being: The reality you engage is determined by the kinds of actions you habitually perform and the material contexts in which you act.

Toward Multiple Ontologies in (Rhetorical) Historiography

My exploration of multiple ontologies begins with the works of Pickering and Mol. Pickering is a sociologist by training, while Mol is a philosopher, but both participate actively in the broadly multidisciplinary STS community. My analysis of their recent theoretical work will focus on Mol's (2002) *The Body Multiple* and Pickering's (2010) *The Cybernetic Brain.* Each of these works explores notions of multiple ontologies and "questions of what the world is like, what sort of entities populate it, how they engage with one another" (Pickering, 2010, p. 17). Both scholars argue that ontologies emerge from practices or performances. The first point here is the idea of "ontologies" that Mol tackles in her earlier (1999) "Ontological Politics." In a move that nicely parallels the decision of some French pain scholars to adopt *douleurs*, Mol pluralizes ontology:

> *Ontologies*: note that. Now the word needs to go in the plural. For, and this is a crucial move, if reality is *done*, if it is historically, culturally and materially *located*, then it is also *multiple*. (p. 71, emphasis in original)

Mol argues that if we can understand things as being manipulated in practices, "if instead of bracketing off practices in which objects are handled,
we foreground them—this has far-reaching effects. Reality multiplies"
(2002, pp. 3–4). Both Mol and Pickering argue that the very idea of a
singular ontology—a basic construct or a set of preconditions for a single reality—is a legacy of modernist and/or positivist notions about the
world. In contrast, each offers thorough and detailed documentation of
how different practices can result in different ontologies. As Mol argues,
"Ontology is not given in the order of things, but . . . instead, *ontologies*
are brought into being, sustained, or allowed to wither away in common,
day to day, sociomaterial practices" (2002, p. 6). Reviewing the theory,
Gad and Jensen (2010) write:

> Reality is manipulated in many ways and does not lie around waiting to be
> glanced at. It does not have "aspects," "qualities," or "essences," which are
> shed light upon by a certain theoretical perspective. However, when doing on-
> tological work, different versions of objects appear. These, in turn, may relate
> and shape partially linked versions of reality. Concepts such as "intervention,"
> "performance," and "enactment" highlight the attempt to approach reality as
> "done" rather than "observed." (p. 71)

Talk about multiple realities may seem bizarre, even counterintuitive,
but it is not a form of anti-realism. Indeed, as Latour argues in *Pandora's
Hope* (1999), this focus on material practices brings a "more realistic realism" (p. 15)—a new materialism—back into the study of science "like
blood through the many vessels now reattached by the clever hands of
the surgeons" (p. 17). The postplural rejection of perspectivalism with its
underlying logic of representation is not a form of anti-realism. In turning
to practices and the term "enactment," Mol, for example, is rejecting the
hegemonic fallacy and its attendant notion of a coherent and unified entity to be called the "social" that could "construct" reality.

The controlling metaphor of both Mol's conception of ontological
"enactment" and Pickering's conception of the "performative" nature of
science is that of the theater and of staging. Mol eschews the troubled
metaphor of "social construction" and says that in site-specific practices,
objects are "done" or "enacted." She uses the theater metaphor to capture the ontological power of practice: "At different times and places
scripts are staged in various ways" (2002, p. 32). She concludes that "when
a disease is being done, we may say that it is *performed* in a specific way"

(2002, p. 32, emphasis in original). Pickering similarly refers to the performative element of cybernetics as "ontological theater" (p. 21). This metaphor has a long history in STS. In their widely cited book, *Leviathan and the Airpump,* Shapin and Shaffer (1985) describe Boyles's experiments with a vacuum pump and his scientific demonstration before an audience of witnesses. Notably, the mechanisms, both human and machine, that did the work of the experiment were concealed beneath the floor. The experiment separated the scientific demonstration before the audience from what Pickering (1995) calls the "mangle of practice," the physical, human, mechanical, political, and economic mangle that performed the experiment and, in Mol's terms, enacted the vacuum. This literal staging produced the scientist as the modest witness separating him- or herself, as well as all the materiality of science, from the results of the experiment, the object known as the vacuum. Similarly, Latour's argument in *Science in Action* (1987) and again in *The Pasteurization of France* (1988) belongs to this performative understanding of scientific practice and the controlling metaphor of theater and enactment.

Mol's exploration of this theory is a detailed ethnographic study of the manifold practices involved in diagnosing, treating, and studying atherosclerosis. In *The Body Multiple,* Mol traces various "atheroscleroses" around a particular hospital in the Netherlands. She explores the different ontologies that emerge from different practices surrounding the same concept. For example, she contrasts the atherosclerosis that is enacted in the vascular surgery clinic from the atherosclerosis that is enacted in the internal medicine clinic. For vascular surgery, atherosclerosis is a *condition* characterized as "encroached vessels" (p. 104). For internal medicine, atherosclerosis is a temporal *process* of "vessel encroachment" (p. 104). In the vascular surgery clinic that Mol describes, surgeons measure the ankle-brachial index (the ratio of blood pressure at the ankle below a blocked leg artery divided by the blood pressure in a healthy arm) using a Doppler device. They examine angiographic images clipped on a light box that show vascular stenoses measured as the amount of vessel lumen lost, roughly the amount of visible encroachment. These technologies define atherosclerosis as a present, measurable condition amenable to surgical intervention and localized and made visible in a specific artery. But in internal medicine, atherosclerosis is a late stage of a gradual process of encroachment, and it concerns the whole vascular system rather than a single artery or a specific location on an artery (p. 122). Internists measure lipoprotein and blood-sugar levels and talk with patients about diet.

In this clinic, atherosclerosis is a matter of future development and of prevention. What each atherosclerosis *is* depends on where it is situated and what practices relate atherosclerosis to other things: instruments, people, complaints, measurements, and so on (p. 54). Different sites of practice enact different diseases. Unlike incommensurable theories of languages, however, these different diseases each have a place in the practice of the other, different clinical practice. Mol's term for this is "layering" (p. 107). For internal medicine, a failed intervention may enact a late stage in which the process becomes a condition and the patient is referred to surgery. Similarly, in the vascular clinic, the accumulation of lipoproteins is an "underlying process" (p. 107) beneath or behind the condition that the surgeons treat. Surgeons and internists treat different diseases, but they also cooperate with each other.

Doing similar theoretical work in *The Cybernetic Brain*, Pickering offers a detailed history of British cybernetics as a critique of modern representational conceptions of science. Pickering organizes his introduction to this history by contrasting two ways to think about the brain, each embedded in different practices of cybernetics. The traditional conception envisions the brain as "an organ of knowledge" (p. 5) possessed of stories, memories, representations of the world, and so on. This "brain" is performed by "GOFAI"—good old-fashioned artificial intelligence (p. 6). By contrast, cybernetics "conceived of the brain as an immediately embodied organ, intrinsically tied into bodily performances" (p. 6). Where the representational brain held knowledge of a preexisting, knowable, and representable world, the cybernetic brain "was not representational but *performative*, as I say, and its role in performance was *adaptation*" (p. 6). Like the surgeons in Mol's study who need information in order to make a decision, the cybernetic brain acts in and on the world. It is what it is by virtue not of its contents but its performance in changing contexts. After reviewing a number of cybernetic experiments, Pickering argues that these experiments "stage" different ontologies that contrast with those of modernist sciences:

> I want to say that cybernetics drew back the veil the modern sciences cast over the performative aspects of the world, including our own being. Early cybernetic machines confront us, instead, with interesting and engaged material performances that do not entail a detour through knowledge. The phrase that runs through my mind at this point is ontological theater. I want to say that cybernetics staged a nonmodern ontology for us in a double sense. (2010, p. 21)

Here Pickering refers to experiments like W. Grey Walter's robotic turtles. Walter developed mechanized turtles designed to interact with and adapt to their environment as part of larger efforts to develop a greater understanding of the workings of the human brain. The very idea that the behavior of a "constructed" machine could offer insight into the "natural" brain does, indeed, stage—to use Pickering's metaphor—a nonmodern ontology. It elides the human/nonhuman dichotomy on which modern ontology (and traditional science) is grounded. Further, the experiments Pickering describes treat the brain as a black box. Rather than opening it up to see what it contains, what representations it has, the cyberneticists manipulated the mechanical brains, testing what they could do. Again, different practices performed or enacted different objects.

Pain Ontologies

I invoke multiple-ontologies theory here because it provides rhetorical-ontological inquiry with a productive alternative to epistemologically focused historiography. The shift to a new materialist approach allows one to interrogate a more mutable conception of scientific practice—one that does not assume that parties with different epistemologies or metaphysics are locked in incommensurable perspectives. Exploring pain medicine through this new materialist rubric, I have identified a multiplicity of pain ontologies, each one nested within the particular practices of health-care providers and researchers. Indeed, this study has identified six different pain ontologies from which different metaphysics and epistemologies of pain emerge. In order to help encapsulate both the multiplicity of pain and its history, I present two different visualizations of these pain ontologies.

My first representation (table 1.1) provides a list of each pain ontology indexed by practical regime and corresponding metaphysics of pain. Concerning this lexicon, Mol is quite physical in her sense of "site of practice" as a "where"—a physical location of a set of practices—understandably, considering her focus on atheroscleroses distributed through different spaces in a hospital. But the idea of specific physical sites of practice is less useful for my inquiry into pain medicine. It would be easy to say that "diagnosis" occurs in the exam room, but that is a somewhat myopic view. Diagnosis occurs equally in the exam room, the laboratory, the library, the Internet, and elsewhere. It is a spatially distributed practice. Additionally, the physical space "exam room" is, in many cases, the exact same location

TABLE 1.1 **Ontologies, emergent metaphysics, and sites of practice in pain medicine**

Pragmatic regimes	Ontology	Metaphysics of pain
Prognosis	Semiotic	Pain as indexical sign
Diagnosis		
Laboratory microscopy	Biochemical	Pain as nociception
Vivisection		
Opiate pharmacology		
Laboratory research	Empirical-discursive	Pain as statistical construct
Computational analysis		
Publication		
Psychotherapy	Cognitive-behavioral	Psychological pain
Multimodal pain management	Nonmodern-practical	Hybrid pain
Pain management theory	Nonmodern-discursive	Phenomenology of suffering

used for both diagnostics and opiate pharmacology, but each practice articulates the exam room to a different set of physical locations. Diagnostic practice articulates itself to all the previously mentioned locations. In contrast, opiate pharmacology articulates the exam room to the same locations as diagnostics, but also to the pharmacy and the patient's medicine cabinet at home. Following Thévnot (2002), I refer to "pragmatic regimes of engagement" or "pragmatic regimes," an all-encompassing term that describes action, practice, habit, and so on. In short, a pragmatic regime of engagement is a way of interacting with the world from which emerges orders of value and agency attributed to people and objects.

Second, for each ontology, I identify an emergent metaphysics of pain. "Emergent" here is not a recapitulation of the two-world problem. Regimes of practice are not sites of physical materiality from which discourse emerges. They are sites of doing, and doing includes the practices of speaking, writing, visualizing, and representing (about which more in chapter 2). In speaking of metaphysical emergence, I capitalize on the understanding of an ontology as the precondition for being. Subsequently, the nature of an object within a given ontological realm would be that object's metaphysics. Different pain ontologies, as they are staged within pragmatic regimes of clinical or medico-scientific practice, result in particular pain metaphysics. The metaphysics of an object is typically articulated (spoken, pronounced) in the formal discourse that surrounds that object, although the metaphysics of the object emerges from the articulations (assemblages) in the regime of practice and the ontology it stages. However, a metaphysics' explicit identification in discourse means that it has traditionally been the first point of analysis for theory succession histories. For example, a metaphysical history of evolutionary theory might trace the shifts from a Lamarckian metaphysics of acquired characteristics to a Darwinian metaphysics of natural selection to a modern synthesis metaphysics that identifies evolution as a function of mutation and genetic drift. In contrast, an ontological history, like the one presented here, begins its analysis with the pragmatic regimes and only subsequently derives emergent ontologies and correlative metaphysics. As I argue in the introduction, a new materialist analysis needs a both/and rather than an either/or approach to inquiry. Thus the metaphysics of pain becomes an important avenue for analysis—as one among many facets of each pain ontology. Indeed, metaphysical issues can sometimes be particularly important when analyzing issues like ontological conflict, as the disputants often articulate ontological differences as metaphysical (theoretical) ones.

My second representation (fig. 1.1) locates the historical emergence of each ontology and identifies key figures and moments in medical history that have contributed to the development of various pain ontologies. Notice that the multiple-ontologies orientation eliminates the possibility of a flat timeline. An epistemologically oriented theory succession approach would locate all of this multiplicity across a single line, with each new theory replacing its predecessor. In contrast, a multiple-ontologies history requires a multilinear expression. I like to think of this visualization as somewhat akin to an evolutionary cladogram. Cladograms are branching-tree diagrams that map speciation and extinction events as traced from provisional origin points. For example, a cladogram of dinosaur evolution begins with a single origin point that splits off pretty immediately into two lines, one that further divides into dozens of species including stegosaurus and triceratops and another that traces the origin of species like the *Brachiosaurus* and *Tyrannosaurus rex*. The branches help the reader identify how closely individual species are related by showing how recently they divided from the prior line. Additionally, some cladograms note the collocations of important geologic or climactic events that might propagate a speciation or an extinction episode. For example, the dinosaur cladogram might indicate the asteroid impact in the late Cretaceous era that prompted their extinction. Similarly, my pain cladogram highlights certain events, such as the publication of the Flexner report, which propagated many changes in U.S. health and medicine.

In the sections that follow, I explore the relationships among pragmatic regimes, emergent ontologies, and metaphysics of pain along various historical lineages as represented in the pain-history cladogram, highlighting

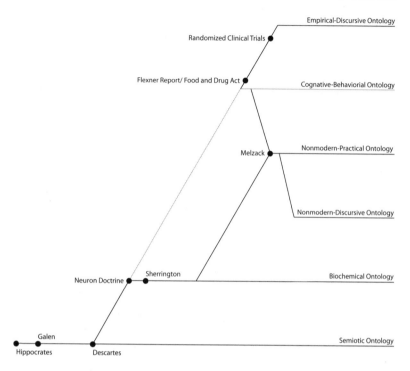

FIGURE 1.1. Pain history. This diagram replicates the logic of multiple ontologies and provides a multilinear conception of pain history. It includes key intellectual figures and important socio-material events that were tremendously transformative.

the value of the multiple-ontologies approach for the analysis of medical history. But the multilinearity of the multiple-ontologies approach precludes a traditional historiographic narrative. I cannot start in antiquity and proceed in a strict temporal order to the present day. Therefore, I focus on one branch at a time—tracing it from origin to present. Then I proceed to the next-most ancient origin point and follow that branch to the present, and so on. This chapter focuses primarily on the first four (historically speaking) ontologies: the semiotic, the biochemical, the empirical-discursive, and the cognitive-behavioral. As the title suggests, the remainder of *The Politics of Pain Medicine* addresses, in more detail, the hybrid ontologies of pain. However, as the hybrid ontologies have emerged out of a combination of appropriation and rejection with regard to the other ontologies, this historical background provides a necessary foundation for understanding the contemporary ontologies.

The Semiotic Pain Ontology

Antiquity

Generally recognized as the father of clinical medicine, Hippocrates (of the famed Hippocratic oath) provides historically oriented scholars of medicine (generally) and scholars of pain medicine (specifically) with a convenient starting point. As is often the case with the prolific authors of ancient Greece, there is a great deal of controversy surrounding which (if any) of the nearly seventy works of medical theory attributed to Hippocrates were actually written by him. Indeed, some scholars suggest that the Hippocratic corpus was written by up to nineteen different people. Still, it is widely accepted that the works of the corpus were all produced by Hippocrates and/or his followers during a relatively short period in Ionian Greece.

It is within the Hippocratic corpus that one can find the origin of the first pain ontology in Western medicine. Among his[3] many theoretical and practical inventions, Hippocrates is responsible for the first formal discourses on the practices of medicine. Though the Hippocratic corpus includes little concerning diagnostics (II.ix)—the contemporary discipline most concerned with the study of signs and symptoms—its discussion of the practices of medical prognosis establishes the first pain ontology: the semiotic ontology. I use the term *semiotic* not in a two-world sense that would suggest that pain was staged as an ephemeral, illusory, or imaginary construct. Rather, I identify the first ontology as a semiotic ontology because the prognostic and diagnostic practices of ancient medicine were keenly focused on the relationship between a sign and its referent. In the absence of readily available laboratory testing and medical imaging, determining how well a patient might fare constituted quite a challenge for the practicing physician. As Hippocrates noted, "He who would make accurate forecasts as to those who will recover, and those who will die, and whether the disease will last a greater or less number of days, must understand all the symptoms thoroughly and be able to appreciate them" (II.xxv). As a part of this practical regime and semiotic ontology, pain must exist primarily as an indexical sign. Pain—in a particular place, of a particular type, of a particular intensity—helps the physician determine prognoses. As Rey (1993) describes Hippocrates's work, "Pain signifies σημίνει (sèmainei), which is certainly not to be taken as an isolated symptom but rather as a part of an overall picture of how the patient looks, what his behavior is like compared to how he generally behaves, his stools, urine, sweat, etc." (p. 20).

In keeping with this approach to pain, Hippocrates's *Prognostics* generally only describes pain as present or absent and by location. For example, in the representative excerpt that follows, the location of pain (in the ear), when combined with the other symptoms, indicates a less than favorable prognosis: "Acute pain of the ear with continuous high fever is dangerous, for the patient is likely to become delirious and die" (II.xxii). This focus on pain as indexical sign was pervasive in ancient medicine. Perhaps the best evidence of this can be found in the work of Roman encyclopedist Aulus Cornelius Celsus (BCE 25–50 CE), which included a broad range of topics from agriculture and oratory to jurisprudence and philosophy. However, only his treatise on medicine (*De Medicina*) survives. Concerning pain, Rey notes:

> In Celsus' approach to medicine, and in the general medical attitude prevalent during Antiquity as a whole, pain had no significance other than its value in announcing specific individual disorders and in providing prognoses; its meaning went no further than such indications, and in consequence, required nothing other than taking the appropriate measures to alleviate it. (1993, p. 26)

The Hippocratic approach to medicine was pervasive in antiquity until the Roman Galen of Pergamon (born CE 129) inaugurated an approach to medicine that remained dominant until early modernity, finally being supplanted by the works of Andreas Vesalius (1548) and William Harvey (1623). Galen was inarguably the most prolific author of antiquity, with more than 600 works in his corpus—although only one-third of them survive today.

Unlike Hippocrates, Galen embraced the need for a thorough approach to diagnostic medicine and subsequently shifted the primary practical regime of engagement, staging the semiotic ontology from which the pain-as-indexical-sign metaphysics emerges. Indeed, his book-length essay *On the Affected Parts* (*De Locis Affectis*) (1976) is entirely devoted to the practices of diagnoses. This is all the more relevant to the case of pain, as Galen's second major section in this work—the section on symptomology—places special emphasis on pain. The following excerpt, which opens the discussion of signs and symptoms, reveals how Galenic medicine reproduces the metaphysics of pain as indexical sign nearly as it had been since Hippocrates:

In regards to the symptoms: Pain is symptomatic of a certain condition or location, cough of others, and in this vomiting, bleeding, loose stools, cramps chills, shivering and delirium. If we distinguish each of these symptoms from the others, then it should be easy to detect what has been defined as good or bad. Examination of every detail will clearly demonstrate that these things truly occur in this manner. (p. 43)

The differences in Galen's approach to pain come not from its basic operating logic but from the focus on diagnostic practices over prognostic. Furthermore, Galen's work is noteworthy for acknowledging and exploring one of pain medicine's primary challenges, even today—properly interpreting patient report:

However, this is difficult to evaluate, since we have to rely on many other persons: either on those who suffer but do not well understand their experiences because their minds are weak, or on those who understand but are unfit to communicate, being totally unable to formulate their suffering in words, since it requires a considerable effort or cannot even be communicated verbally. Consequently, a person who wants to describe each type of pain should have experienced it personally, should also be a physician and able to express it to others, and should observe it with understanding while suffering, and with his mental powers intact. (p. 51)

Here one can see the early stages of a problem that will long plague pain medicine in a variety of ontologies. Physicians can only access pain through patient report, and patient report is by definition subjective and variant. This is an issue of continued frustration for physicians who see pain as semiotic and therefore already one step removed from the supposedly more real mechanisms of injury. This two-world juxtaposition of subjective patient report and objective mechanism of injury comes with great cost for patients with difficult-to-assess conditions, an issue that will be addressed at great length in chapters 3 and 4.

The Rise of Modernity

Though the effects are delayed, the rise of empirical method in early modernity constitutes the locus of the first bifurcation in my pain ontologies cladogram. The new pragmatic regimes of engagement inaugurated by modernity will be interrogated in the sections that follow. However, unlike theory succession accounts of scientific revolution, this change in the practices of pain science and management did not result in a new theory that supplanted the previous regime. Indeed, an incarnation of the semiotic ontology and its corresponding metaphysics of pain remains extant even today. So while I will save for later my discussion of the new discourse that arose out of modernity, this section will explore the effects of modernity on the discourse of pain as indexical sign.

As Foucault (1970/1966) describes it in *The Order of Things*—his archaeology of the transformation from the classical to the modern episteme—one of the fundamental features of the shift into modernity was a change in status for language:

> Language began to fold in upon itself, to acquire its one particular density, to deploy a history, an objectivity, and laws of its own. It became one object of knowledge among others, on the same level as living beings, wealth and value, and history of events and men. (p. 296)

This objectification of language spawned new disciplines of linguistic inquiry—specifically, philology and a new semiology. This semiology provided the backdrop for a more nuanced approach to pain as indexical sign. It challenged the direct indexicality of the previous age and began a project of taxonomy that identified and classified various forms of pain and subsequently determined their referents. During this era, "the essential question for the physician was to know whether a particular type of pain could allow one to determine that a given part of the body was affected and/or that a particular illness had befallen the patient" (Rey, 1993, p. 97).

This developing pain taxonomy was coupled with a semiotic approach to other signs and symptoms and catalogued in diagnostic manuals. Pain as indexical sign was now understood in relation to the other common signs such as "pulse, urine, respiration, tongue, face, etc." (Rey, p. 94). This approach to pain further relegated pain to an issue of secondary concern for the practicing physician. For example, in the first entry in the *Encyclopaedic Index of Medicine and Surgery* (1882), "Abdomen, Contusions and Wounds of," pain is the *sixth* symptom listed for an ailment that might have resulted from any of the following causes: "blows, falls, the passage of wheels, pressure between opposing forces, wounds with knives, razors, daggers, sabres, bayonets, horns of animals, gun and pistol shot wounds, etc." (Bermingham, 1882, p. 5). Specifically, the text states that in cases of abdominal contusions or wounds:

There is pain, sudden in character, and probably attended by swelling, the result of effused blood, and probably indicated by a dent in, or by a marked separation of the torn ends of the muscle. The pain is increased on motion to such an extent that the movements of the body may be almost impossible for a time. Contusion with rupture of viscera is characterized by sudden, sometimes excessive, pain, great depression, intense anxiety, rapid pulse, vomiting, [and] great thirst. (p. 5)

In order to help the practicing clinician make use of these semiotic taxonomies, diagnostic textbooks from the nineteenth century include primers on inductive logic.

Nineteenth-century clinicians were taught to consider all the signs and their categories and in so doing perform a series of inferences that would lead to diagnoses. Barclay's (1862) *Manual of Medical Diagnosis* includes an excellent example of this type of discourse:

All true diagnosis is ultimately based upon inductions separately framed out of clinical and pathological investigations and experiments. By careful and repeated observation, we have succeeded, with every appearance of truth, in associating certain phenomena observed during life with particular lesions found after death; and these form the first step in our progress. . . . In so far as we are able to correctly interpret symptoms, and to trace out in connection with them a real change of structure or of function which affords an adequate explanation of their presence, in so far are we prepared to form a correct diagnosis. (p. 29)

From the nineteenth century to the present, incorporation into the current practical regimes is the only real change for the pain's semiotic ontology. The taxonomies are refined and complexified; the logics shift.

Contemporary diagnostic manuals treat pain in much the same fashion as those of the nineteenth century. Pain is considered as one sign among many in the fashioning of diagnostic pronouncement. For comparison, see the current approach to abdominal pain in *French's Differential Diagnosis* (2005):

A common and extremely important clinical problem is the patient who presents with acute abdominal pain. This may be referred all over the abdominal wall, but here we shall consider those patients who present pain localized to a particular part of the cavity. The causes are legion, and it is a useful exercise to summarize the organs that may be implicated together with the pathological

processes pertaining to them so that the clinician can consider the possibilities
in a logical manner. (Kinirons & Ellis, 2005, p. 1)

As can be seen, this passage follows the organization of the previously
cited 1862 manual almost exactly. Though pain is listed as the first symptom, the text proceeds from symptom to a list of underlying causes.
Though the contemporary list offers a greater variety of "pathological
processes" than the mostly brute injuries of the 1862 text, overall it is
highly similar. What has changed is the logic for unifying the various signs
of diagnoses. No longer are medical students given lessons in inductive
logic. The primacy of logic in diagnostic assessment has been supplanted
by a focus on evidence-based medicine (EBM), and the primary logic
of EBM is statistics.[4] Diagnostics is now a process of comparing the observed (or experimentally derived) signs and symptoms with statistical
tables that help the clinician determine the additive probability of each
new symptom. Contemporary diagnostics manuals are filled with formu-
las and probabilistic discussions like the following from McGee's (2007)
Evidence-Based Physical Diagnosis:

> Pretest probability is the probability of disease (i.e., prevalence) before appli-
> cation of the results of a physical finding. Pretest probability is the starting
> point for all clinical decisions. For example, the clinician may know that a cer-
> tain physical finding shifts the probability of a disease upward 40%, but this in-
> formation alone is unhelpful unless the clinician also knows the starting point:
> If the pretest probability for a particular diagnosis was 50%, the finding is diag-
> nostic (i.e., post-test probability 50% + 40% = 90%); if the pretest probability
> was only 10%, the finding is less helpful, because the probability of disease is
> still the flip of a coin (i.e., post-test probability 10% + 40% = 50%). (p. 4)

Although it has been co-opted by the statistical regime of EBM, pain as
indexical sign is an extant metaphysics with no indication of impending
extinction. In fact, pain's status as indexical sign was further enfranchised
in the early 2000s when it was dubbed the "fifth vital sign" by professional
organizations, hospital administrative bodies, and, in some cases, legal
mandate. Now joined to pulse, respiration, temperature, and blood pressure, pain is widely considered an essential part of determining the basic
health of a patient. So while the practices of medicine have been sub-
divided into a complex and bewildering concatenation of subdisciplines,
each with internal logics of their own, the semiotic pain ontology has been
relegated to diagnostics.

The Biochemical Ontology

In order to explore how pain has been realized within these emergent sub-specialties, this history of pain must return to the advent of the modern era—the epoch responsible for the scientification of medicine and its subsequent differentiation into subdisciplines. The rise of modernity, its new scientific model, and the concomitant epistemological transformation that occurred in Western thought was, as is well known, broadly influential on all areas of intellectual life. The new methodological tools offered by empiricism created a substantially new approach to knowledge that has been well documented by history, philosophy, sociology, and rhetoric of science. The epistemological, methodological, and ontological transformation that inaugurated the modern era began in the early 1600s and had nearly immediate impacts on medical science. Indeed, it is widely argued in historical studies of science and philosophy that the new episteme was initialized by either Francis Bacon's 1620 publication of the *Novum Organon* or René Descartes's *Discourse on Method* in 1637. Likewise, William Harvey is considered the first scholar of modern medical science. As Rey describes it:

> In the 17th century, mankind's knowledge took a great leap forward thanks to Harvey's discovery of the circulation of the blood, which he described in his *Exercitatio anatomica de motu cordis et sanguinis in anima*, published in 1628. Indeed, this work was a turning point in the history of medicine, because it would allow physiologists and doctors alike to gradually break free from the legacy of Galen. They would become free to develop new methods of investigation and to dare uphold that their observations and deductions could be more accurate than those handed down from Antiquity. However, it should be added that this analytical attitude, which had begun to take form in the previous century, also benefitted from the success of the revolution in physics and astronomy which came about as a result of new explanations of the universe formulated in terms of mathematical principles. (1993, p. 71)

While the rise of modernity has been discussed by innumerable texts and authors, I have found the discussions offered by Foucault and Latour to be most informative when it comes to understanding this epoch's ontological emergences. While Latour, following the lead of many, focuses on Descartes and the *Cogito,* Foucault's *Order of Things* and *Archaeology of Knowledge* interrogate the establishment of the modern episteme as half of a two-part transformation wherein modernity was brought forth through an intervening "classical episteme." As this term suggests, Foucault's historiography is not explicitly new materialist; neither, for that matter, is Latour's discussion of the rise of modernity. Nevertheless, both thinkers have been instrumental in the shift toward new materialisms. As such, it is not too much of a stretch to reinterpret their discussions of the rise of modernity within a new materialist idiom.

As Foucault notes, the classical seventeenth-century episteme broke from the prior scholastic tradition by shifting away from the traditional focus on language (dialectic) as path to knowledge toward the adoption of a new regime dominated by the logics of the will-to-truth and the will-to-knowledge:

> A will to knowledge emerged which, anticipating its present content, sketched out a schema of possible, observable, measurable and classifiable objects; and a will to knowledge which imposed upon the knowing subject—in some ways taking precedence over all experience—a certain position, a certain viewpoint, and a certain function (look rather than read, verify rather than comment). . . . (Foucault, 1972, p. 218)[5]

While Foucault ultimately situates Descartes as a transitional figure located between the classical (will-to-truth) and modern (will-to-knowledge) epistemes, he recognizes Descartes's work as pivotal in the series of transformations that eventually culminates in the modernity (1970/1966, p. 52). Indeed, Descartes's work in the *Discourse on Method* is (in)famous for the establishment of the two-world problem and its correlative dualisms. As Latour notes in *Pandora's Hope* (1999), Descartes's separation of mind and body resulted in the establishment of a "brain- [or mind-] in-a-vat"—Latour's metaphor for a disconnected mind seeking absolute certainty (p. 4). As is well known, Descartes used this separation between mind and body as a foundation for the separation between the mind and the world outside, establishing an epistemology predicated on "the notion of a world 'out there' to which a mind-in-a-vat tries to get access by establishing some safe correspondence between words and states of affairs" (Latour, 1999, p. 113).

Despite the epistemological tenor of Latour's and Foucault's analysis, their insights into Descartes and the rise of empiricism have as much (if not more) to do with doing than knowing. Indeed, Descartes's most famous treatise concerns method, and Foucault's analysis of the will-to-knowledge focuses on how the methodologies of scientific practice lead to technological activity. Certainly these methods have profound epistemological ramifications. Nevertheless, the unyielding epistemological orientation of Foucault's and Latour's analyses are products of their time—an era dominated by epistemological angst as a result of the postmodern reification of the two-world problem. And here again, we see that the two-world problem simultaneously has profound impacts on both pain science and humanistic/cultural studies.

With this new methodological foundation, Descartes began his task of developing a new metaphysics and new practical regimes of engagement for interrogating this new "world out there." And, of course, this resulted in one of the most mechanistic approaches to natural philosophy ever devised. This history is relevant for two very important reasons. First, it was this mechanism that provided the beginning for the new scientifically grounded approach to medicine such as the one used by Harvey. As Rey (1993) describes it:

> In this context where Mechanism was triumphing in the natural sciences, medicine tried to envisage the human body as a complex machine which could be compared to an ensemble of ropes, levers, and pulleys. It tied reason to "geometric fashion" i.e. by rigorously stringing together all its propositions and accepting only those that which could be proven. (pp. 71–72)

Second, this rather abstract discussion concerning methodological transformation is critical to understanding the development of pain ontologies. The first firmly established departure from the semiotic pain ontology was not only predicated on Cartesian methodology—it was literally authored by René Descartes himself.

Pain Objectified

In the wake of the modern methodological/ontological shift, for the first time since antiquity a new pain ontology emerged. It is highly distinct from the semiotic ontology in that it repositioned pain as a metaphysical object in its own right rather than a means of crossing the epistemological-metaphysical division. No longer was pain primarily a semiotic phenomenon; pain itself now became an object of study. As Rey (1993) notes:

[Pain's] specificity as an object of scientific interest went unrecognized for a long time and for a variety of frequently contradictory reasons: deemed the inevitable accompaniment of illness, pain was usually acknowledged and then relegated to a place of secondary importance, rather than studied for its own intrinsic qualities. (p. 6)

Given this new order of pain objectification, it seems only fitting that one of the first and most persuasive treatments of pain as object was offered by Descartes. One of his many endeavors after the publication of the *Discourse of Method* was a new science of anatomy and physiology—more specifically, the physiology of pain and sensation. Not only did Descartes's development of pain theory follow his establishment of the *Cogito*, it was likely based on it. As mentioned in the outset of this chapter, he was the first thinker to propose the theory of pain transmission—that is, a theory that describes how pain impulses or signals are propagated from the skin to the mind. This is appropriate, however, since such a theory would have been impossible before the two-world hypothesis and its correlative stipulation that the mind and body were separate things. Descartes described his model with a paired diagram (fig. 1.2) and textual explanation that thoroughly demonstrate his commitment to a mechanistic understanding of the world and the human body:

> Thus, for example, if fire A is near foot B, the tiny parts of this fire—which as you know move very rapidly—have sufficient force to move with them the area of skin that they touch, and in this way they pull the tiny fibre *cc* which you see attached to it, and simultaneously open the entrance to pore *de*, located opposite the point where this fibre terminates [in the brain]: just as when you pull on one end of a cord you cause a bell hanging on the other end to ring at the same time. (1662/2004, p.117)

Interestingly, this passage reads more like a contemporary instruction manual than an anatomy or physiology text. Of Descartes's model, Řey writes (1993):

> This model of pain was one among several prominent competing theories in the classical and early modern eras. While its immediate impact on medical science of Descartes's era is unclear it was highly influential in Descartes's developing thought and the theories of his followers. Most importantly perhaps, it was Descartes work on pain and sensation that led him to develop his theory of the

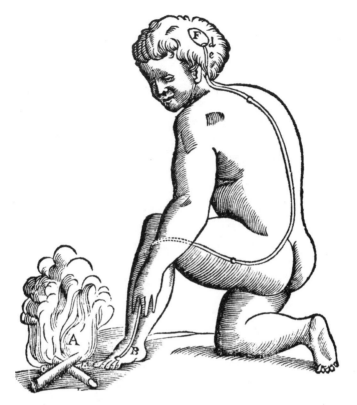

FIGURE 1.2. Descartes's transmission model of pain. While this model, the first of its kind, was not widely accepted during Descartes's time, it would eventually become the cornerstone for one of the most persuasive pain-qua-object ontologies.

pineal gland—the neurological structure which links soul and body. (Rey, 1993, pp. 74–75)

However, I highlight Descartes's theory of pain not so much for its influence among his contemporaries but rather for its influence in twentieth-century pain science and medicine. As Morris (1991) notes:

Descartes's rope-pull model of pain is a direct predecessor of the organic model developed in the mid-nineteenth century. Doctors and researchers adhering to the organic model now talk about nociceptive impulses and endorphins rather than about filaments and animal spirits, but the basic idea is the same. They view pain as the result of a universal, internal mechanism that sends a signal from the injury to the brain. (p. 271)

The continued importance and influence of this model to contemporary approaches to pain can be seen from the fact that it is widely cited, as noted in the introduction, for having gotten it essentially "right." (See Melzack, 1973, p. 126; Melzack & Wall, 1982, pp. 149–150; and Fishman & Berger, 2000, p. 9, for a few prominent examples.) Of course, pain clinicians and researchers who trace their work back to Descartes typically neglect the passage immediately following the preceding description of pain transmission. Indeed, they seem little interested in Descartes's description of the human response to painful stimuli:

> Now when the entrance to this pore or small tube *de* is opened this way, the animal spirits carry from cavity *F* enter and are carried through it, some to the muscles that serve to pull the foot away from the fire, and some to the muscles that make the hands move and the whole body turn in order to protect itself. (1662/2004, p. 117)

Pain as Nociception

Despite Descartes's early foray into pain science, pain's biochemical ontology wouldn't be fully realized until the twentieth century—and the staging of the metaphysics of pain as nociception. While Descartes was certainly responsible for the emergence of the biochemical pain ontology, it would take several centuries of engagement with laboratory practices before a stable pain metaphysics within that ontology would emerge. Despite this lag, the pain as nociception metaphysics is a product of the biochemical ontology was still grounded in Descartes's notion of pain transmission. Indeed, Rey's (1993) chapter heading for the nociceptive model of pain is "Communication Strategies: The Approach to Pain During the First Half of the 20th Century." As she further explains:

> A primary preoccupation [of this era in pain science] concerned the pathway connecting one point to another, the time it took to travel along it, and the various states and transmission relays along the way. Research on pain was dominated by problems of communication, speed, and efficiency. (p. 263)

While communication models of pain had (as evidenced by Descartes) been discussed at a much earlier date, the intervening establishment of the neuron doctrine solidified transmission as *the* mechanism of pain physiology. Although Descartes may have pioneered the modern approach to bodies passing impulses to the brain, medical science at large was dubious until they came to an agreement on the underlying mechanism of information transmission. First proposed by Santiago Ramón y Cajal and finalized by Heinrich Wilhelm Gottfried von Waldeyer-Hartz, the neuron doctrine established that nervous impulses are transmitted via electrochemical propagation along a network of closely aligned task-specific cells dubbed "neurons." Waldeyer-Hartz published his seminal work on the subject, "Ueber einige neuere Forschungen im Gebiete der Anatomie des Centralnervensystems" (About some new researches in the field of anatomy of the central nervous system), in the journal *Deutsche medicinische Wochenschrift* in 1891.

This work provided a foundation for contemporary neurophysiology and exposed medical scientists more broadly to the practical regime of engagement centered around laboratory microscopy for neuroanatomy. The images resulting from these practices came in the form of sketches drawn from Waldeyer-Hartz's microscopic observations and displayed how neurological impulses could originate in a single neuron or cluster of neurons and be transmitted along the peripheral nervous system (PNS) to the central nervous system (CNS). This work helped to codify the distinction between PNS (body) and CNS (brain) that began as early as Descartes (albeit under different nomenclature) and continues strongly into the present.

Building on the foundations provided by the neuron doctrine, physiological researchers built new theories of pain much more rapidly than before. As Rey notes in the introduction to her *History of Pain*, pain research has often found itself at an odd multidisciplinary nexus: "Historically speaking, knowledge about pain has usually been gathered within the framework of the strained—frequently broken, and then reestablished—relationship between experimental physiology and clinical medicine" (p. 7). With the establishment of the neuron doctrine in the end of the nineteenth and the beginning of the twentieth century, the study of pain was codified into a thoroughly modernist science. As such, it became capable of wielding considerable power over both experimental physiology and clinical medicine. Ultimately, the neuron doctrine is an integral part of the development of contemporary metaphysics of pain physiology and the reliance on opioid pharmacology that dominates contemporary clinical practice. However, before any of this could happen, pain researchers needed to take neuron theory and apply its tenets to the study of pain. Historical treatments of medicine (whether by historians or physicians) broadly credit C. S. Sherrington, a neurophysiologist from Cambridge, with the identification of the neuromechanical means of pain transmission. Rey (1993) goes so far as to suggest that even though the bulk of Sherrington's research on pain mechanisms was published before 1910, he "really belongs to contemporary science due to the nature of his theories" (p. 279). Rhetorically speaking, this is probably an accurate assessment—Sherrington's description of pain neurophysiology hardly differs from those of contemporary authorship. Indeed, Sherrington's research not only founded what I have identified as the pain as nociception metaphysics, but it also earned him both an English knighthood in 1922 and the Nobel Prize in Physiology or Medicine in 1932.

As a physiologist of his era, Sherrington used the practical regimes of laboratory science then available—a combination of microscopy and vivisection. Indeed, his groundbreaking article that established the pain as nociception metaphysics (1903) used the cold, detached language of science to describe a research methodology that involved intentionally inflicting pain on laboratory dogs that had been subjected to surgical mutilation:

> In the "spinal" dog (e.g. after exsection of a short piece, a segment, from the posterior cervical region of the cord) if the skin underneath and between the toe-pads and cushion of the hind-foot be pressed or stretched, a sudden forcible extension of the limb is evoked. This is especially the case if at the time of stimulation the limb be resting flexed at hip and knee. (p. 39)

While, thankfully, the spinal dog as exemplar animal in pain research has been largely abandoned, spinal rats (subjected to similar protocols) are still a staple of neurophysiological research. Even though the ethics of these experiments are broadly questioned,[6] the experiments themselves are largely credited with providing medical science with true knowledge of the neurophysiology of pain. In Sherrington's case, they led to the verification of both transmission theory and specificity theory (the idea that there are specific nervous fibers that transmit specific types of information—for example, pain or pressure or pleasure).

Sherrington's aforementioned 1903 piece published in the *Journal of Physiology* provided the first objective evidence of pain-specific transmission fibers:

> I have elsewhere put forward a view that there has been evolved in the skin "a special sense of its own injuries." There is considerable evidence that the skin is

provided with a set of nerve-endings whose specific office it is to be amenable
to stimuli that do the skin injury, stimuli that in continuing to act would injure
it still further. These nerve-endings when still connected with the sensorium
(using that term simply to mean the neural machinery to which consciousness
is adjunct) on excitation evoke skin pain. (p. 40)

Following this paragraph, Sherrington coined the term *nocicipient* for
pain transmission fibers (p. 41). Though this variant of the term never
really caught on, it provided the foundation for the publication of a collection of Sherrington's lectures in 1906 that firmly established not only
the theory but also the jargon of pain as nociception. As Sherrington describes it, "Reflexes initiated from a species of receptor apparatus that
may be termed *'noci-ceptive'* appear to particularly dominate the majority of the final common paths issuing from the spinal cord" (p. 226).
Sherrington's (1906) work in *Integrative Action of the Nervous System* (the
aforementioned lecture collection) went on to theorize the mechanisms
of nociception and modes of evaluating nociception in terms of intensity
of stimulus.

In so doing, Sherrington manages to further divorce physical pain from
the mind and describe how noxious stimuli can produce certain electrochemical responses in nociceptive fibers that, if of sufficient intensity, may
be labeled by the conscious mind as "pain":

In the simpler sensations we experience from various kinds of stimuli applied
to our skin there can be distinguished those of touch, of could, of warmth, and
of pain. . . . In evidence of this it is urged that mechanical stimuli applied at
certain places excite sensations which from their very threshold upward possess
unpleasantness, and as the intensity of the stimulus is increased, culminate in
"physical pain." (1906, p. 226)

This increased mind/body separation and subsequent focus on intensity is
a perfect corollary to the biochemical ontology from which it was staged
and further was (and is) so universally accepted that it was heralded almost seventy years later as a beautiful theory "that is rightfully considered
to be a biological principle or law" (Melzack, 1973, p. 133). This accolade
is perhaps all the more impressive as Melzack (about which more later)
is the architect of one of the hybrid pain metaphysics that seeks to supplant the rubrics of pain as nociception.

The biochemical ontology and subsequent metaphysics of pain as nociception has turned out to be highly generative—in both the practical

and rhetorical senses. The transmission and specificity doctrines on which nociception is based coordinate seamlessly with the vast material enterprises surrounding opiate pharmacology. Indeed, opiates—a technology long considered a mystery—have only recently begun to "make sense" to the medical and pharmacological communities in that they can now be understood as hindrances to nociception. This calibration between nociception and pharmacology is critical from a practical perspective as it has produced a new regime of medicine that until recently was almost universally embraced by patient and physician alike. Certainly, the impact of morphine on medical practices from the battlefield to the hospital has been well documented by a cornucopia of sources. The pain as nociception metaphysics inaugurated a new era of medical and pharmaceutical research aimed at understanding and controlling the transmission of nervous signals.

Pain's Empirical-Discursive Ontology

As would be expected, pain's relocation under the biochemical ontology of contemporary medicine was part of a broader project of the scientification of health care. This process was well documented by Foucault's *Birth of the Clinic,* which charts the appropriation of nosology (the study of diseases), and Paul Starr's (1982) *Social Transformation of American Medicine,* which explores (among other things) the professionalization and legitimization of American medicine through an alliance with science. The shift in medicine's privileged, practical regimes of engagement, from clinical art to empirical science, was critical in establishing both the biochemical and empirical-discursive ontologies. Indeed, the development of the new empirical-discursive ontology—and its attendant metaphysics of pain as statistical construct—is part of a long process in medicine's evolution that began with the establishment of the logic of the gaze was aided (in America) by the publication of the Flexner report, and became solidified by the advent of EBM. Of course, there are entire books dedicated to each of these "events" in medical history, and there is no way I can offer an adequate treatment of any one of them within the confines of this chapter. However, a brief acknowledgment of the contexts and effects of each of these moments is critical to the task of providing an adequate background for the pain as statistical construct metaphysics.

Foucault's *Birth of the Clinic* is famous for its archaeology of clinical medicine. This work traces the transformation of medicine into medical science as it occurred in eighteenth- and nineteenth-century France.[7] Though Foucault traces this transformation back to many sources, the proscription to relocate clinical medicine under the empirical practices of observational science was perhaps most succinctly and aptly put by Lyons physician Marc-Antoine Petit: "One must, as far as possible, make science ocular" (quoted in Foucault, 1973/1963, p. 108). As Foucault notes, this mandate that clinical medicine be subsumed under the logic of the gaze was linked to a great variety of medical practices and used as a foundation for clinical authority:

> So many powers, from the slow illumination of obscurities, the ever-prudent reading of the essential, the calculation of times and risks, to the mastery of the heart and the majestic confiscation of paternal authority, are just so many forms in which the sovereignty of the gaze gradually establishes itself—the eye that knows and decides, the eye that governs. (p. 108)

This environment where "for the clinic all truth is sensible truth" (Foucault, 1973/1963, p. 148) was readily embraced by both the French and American medical establishments and inaugurated a great shift in medical theory and practice. As Foucault notes, this transformation was expedited in France by the establishment of a somewhat unified clinical system. Without this sociopolitical mechanism, it would be some time more before the new approach to medicine was broadly accepted in America. Certainly, it should be noted that "gaze" is, in some ways, a perspectivalist metaphor, and, as such, it focuses on the empirical and metaphysical. Nevertheless, such a powerful construct should not be discarded. Thus, in a manner not inconsistent with Foucault, I use the term "gaze" as a way of talking about the metadiscursive elements of medico-scientific ontology. That is, medical scientists engage in certain practical regimes microscopy, neuroimaging, clinical observation, and so on. These practices stage an empirical-discursive ontology—that is, an ontology dominated by representational practices both in the laboratory (the creation of neuroimages, microscopy slides, and so on) and in scholarly publications. These practitioners use the logic of the gaze to justify their practices and insights. More than that, however, gazing is a form of doing. The formal and ritualistic-looking practices of laboratory science are what take center stage in an ontological account, and they are central to my discussion of the discursive-empirical ontology of pain.

Following the rise of the gaze in the late nineteenth and early twentieth century, the American Medical Association (AMA)—the premier organization for allopathic physicians—launched a new campaign of purification designed to limit the field of competition by challenging the validity of alternate schools of health and medicine, including osteopathy, homeopathy, midwifery, and so on. The AMA enlisted the aid of the "independent" Carnegie Foundation for Advancement in Teaching to investigate the state of American medical education. The Carnegie Foundation then, around 1906, tapped Abraham Flexner—a young educator with political connections—to conduct a survey of American medical education. This study resulted in the famous book-length report *Bulletin Number Four*, published in 1910. In this treatise, Flexner censures most American medical schools for great failures in both physician education and protecting the public good. More specifically, as Starr notes, "As Flexner saw it, a great discrepancy had opened up between medical science and medical education. While science had progressed, education had lagged behind" (p. 120).

Essentially, Flexner condemned any school that had not adopted a scientific approach to medicine (that is, one grounded in the practical regimes of laboratory science) and in so doing accepted the sovereignty of the gaze. Indeed, in *Bulletin Number Four*, Flexner argues that medicine had entered a new age of scientific accuracy dominated by the primacy of observation and experimentation:

> The third era [modern medicine] is dominated by the knowledge that medicine is part and parcel of modern science. The human body belongs to the animal world. It is put together of tissues and organs, in their structure, origin, and development not essentially unlike what the biologist is otherwise familiar with; it grows, reproduces itself, decays, according to general laws. It is liable to attack by hostile physical and biological agencies; now struck with a weapon, again ravaged by parasites. The normal course of bodily activity is a matter of observation and experience; the best methods of combating interference must be learned in much the same way. (p. 53)

Following the clinical and laboratory practices outlined by Foucault's archaeology, Flexner's report places tremendous importance on the observational and experimental practices of the empirical sciences. Indeed, in his proscribed approach to medical education, scientific training must be considered a prerequisite for medical knowledge and practice. Not only do physicians need an understanding of the basic clinical sciences such as "anatomy, physiology, [and] physiological chemistry," they also need continuing education in more advanced knowledge—that is, those of "experimental physiology, pathology, and bacteriology" (Flexner, 1910, p. 24).

Additionally, this knowledge involves both basic precepts and theoretical insights, and it must also include education in the practices of experiment and observation and the attendant technologies of an increasingly powerful gaze:

> Succeed as he might, however, [the physician's] possibilities in the way of reducing, differentiating, and interpreting phenomena, or significant aspects of phenomena, were abruptly limited by his natural powers. These powers are nowadays easily enough transcended. The self-registering thermometer, the stethoscope, the microscope, the correlation of observed symptoms with the outgivings of chimerical analysis and biological experimentation, enormously extend the physician's range. He perceives more speedily and more accurately what he is actually dealing with; he knows with far greater assurance the merits or the limitations of the agents which he is in position to invoke. (p. 20)

This report arrived amid a perfect storm of economic decline, governmental regulation, and AMA purification, and the result was a massive reduction in the number of American medical schools (Starr, 1982, p. 118). Those that survived this period of purification were those who accepted regulation and accreditation by the AMA and modified their curricula in accordance with medical science and the sovereignty of the gaze. And as Starr has explained, this educational transformation resulted in a similar change within the broader culture of American medicine. Specifically, "As American medical education became increasingly dominated by scientists and researchers, doctors came to be trained according to the values and standards of academic specialists" (p. 123).

In the very same year (1906) that the AMA commissioned the Carnegie Foundation to start its investigation of American medical schools, President Theodore Roosevelt signed into law the Pure Food and Drug Act that provided for the establishment of what has become one of the United States' most prominent and powerful regulatory agencies—the Food and Drug Administration (FDA). The establishment of the FDA arose out of some of the very same sociopolitical issues that led to Flexner's work. Specifically, the heightened sense of competition in American health care following the Civil War created an environment where various professional organizations lobbied for economically advantageous regulation and legislation. As Cooper (2006) notes in his chapter for the FDA's (sometimes self-aggrandizing) centennial history:

> Before the [Civil War], the professions of medicine and pharmacy had begun to separate, as more highly trained physicians lobbied for state statutes to bar pharmacists from diagnosing. In turn, better educated pharmacists sought to eliminate competition from grocers and other uneducated formulators and dispensers of "patent" medicines. . . . Physicians' and pharmacists' attacks on each other, coupled with newspaper attacks on incompetence and both professions, generated public concern about drugs. Such attacks and concerns have ample basis, for neither medicine nor pharmacy had a firm scientific basis. (p. 30)

Of course, the response to this climate of combined professional organization and consumer outcry was the aforementioned establishment of the FDA. While the FDA of the early twentieth century vigorously pursued many of the shared goals of the current FDA, there is actually little similarity between the organization of the past and the present. Early on, the FDA functioned more as a branch of law enforcement and routinely raided pharmaceuticals' manufacturing plants and distribution centers, seizing improperly labeled or marketed drugs. Though the FDA underwent a number of transformations in its evolution, the most important for pain as statistical construct metaphysics was Congress's 1962 amendment to what was now known as the Federal Food, Drug and Cosmetic Act, which would profoundly revolutionize the science and practice of medicine. The law's new provision required that all pharmaceuticals marketed in the United States should demonstrate safety and efficacy through "adequate and well-controlled investigations." Though this phrase was tailored somewhat haphazardly in an effort to avoid specific definitions concerning evidentiary sufficiency, it has become the cornerstone of EBM (Crout, Vodra, & Werble, 2006, p. 159).

The late sixties and early seventies marked the systemization of the clinical trials approach to medicine. With the public outcry following the thalidomide disaster and similar events, new regulations were enacted worldwide to ensure that human pharmaceuticals would not be distributed without documented safety and efficacy.[8] In 1975, the World Health Organization (WHO) published an international mandate outlining the proper procedures for pharmaceutical evaluation, and these procedures still form the backbone of contemporary pharmacological research. Specifically, the WHO outlined a multistage, progressive process for pharmaceutical evaluation. Only when basic chemical testing has been completed can investigators move on to research in animal models and finally humans:

> When a compound is found to have interesting pharmacological activity, it is investigated in depth. Before starting this work it is essential to characterize the chemical and physical properties of the new compound. The substance is then subjected to a wide range of pharmacological tests and animals to detect any effects that may be of therapeutic use. Many compounds are rejected at this stage, but those that survive are further investigated to determine there are pharmacodynamic and pharmacokinetic properties and to assess their toxicity. When adequate data are available, early studies are initiated in man and, if successful, are followed by controlled therapeutic trials. (WHO Scientific Group, 1975, p. 10)

For the WHO it's "controlled therapeutic trials" and for the 1965 FDA revision it was "well-controlled investigations," and eventually these practices would come to be known under the broad rubric of randomized controlled trials (RCTs). RCTs are the cornerstone of EBM—the contemporary benchmark for scientific medicine. As Dunn and Everett note in *Clinical Biostatistics* (1995), RCTs are the means by which we cope with the fact that "the distinct feature of modern science is *skepticism*: we are no longer prepared to take the pronouncements of authority on trust. We ask for evidence and we wish to evaluate the claims of experts (whether they be scientists, clinicians or politicians)" (p. 2, emphasis in original).

Indeed, RCTs are the strategic realization of the scientific demands placed on the American medical community by the Flexner report. RCTs provide contemporary scientists with a rigorous approach to observation and experiment:

> The scientific approach to medicine demands that we question claims about health and illness by recourse to observation and experiment. We check claims against the empirical evidence. In order to deal to do this, we need to be able to understand the nature of evidence (*the data*) and to the way in which it has been collected and presented. (Dunn & Everett, 1995, p. 2)

To this cursory gloss of the history of the rise of EBM and the hegemony of the RCT, I must add only one additional note. While RCTs and EBM began in the early 1970s, they were not fully realized until the late 1980s and early 1990s. At its heart, contemporary EBM is a statistical discipline, and its establishment required the promulgation of computational research practices adequate to the computational demands. Tellingly, Dunn and Everett open their textbook by quoting Florence Nightingale: "To understand God's thoughts we must study statistics, for those are the measure of his purpose" (p. 1).

In a medical tradition dominated by RCTs and EBM, pain needed to be disciplined under the rubric of statistics. But, of course, this presents clinicians with an enormous problem. Nociception is not directly measurable in clinical patients—as it would require vivisection and thus violate the Hippocratic "do no harm" edict. But the patient's report of pain is inherently subjective and therefore untrustworthy. "Discipline"—in the Foucauldian sense—really is the operative term when it comes to the statistics of pain. And here we have one of the key insights of an ontological historiography that might be elided by other approaches. The laboratory practices of contemporary medical science stage an empirical-discursive ontology. That is, they only recognize certain types of phenomena as real. A patient complaint does not fall under that rubric. Complaints are not present in the ontological staging of this practical regime of engagement. However, pain researchers do not have any choice but to access that information in some fashion. Therefore, in order to fold pain reports into the logic of statistics, clinicians and researchers needed to develop instruments to discipline the patient's report. Subsequently, researchers have come up with investigational practices with which patients are allowed to express their pain but that codify those expressions within the empirical ontology—that render those expressions amenable to statistical evaluation.

One of the simplest and most readily available is the numeric pain rating scale (NPRS). When pain is assessed using the NPRS, patients are simply asked to quantify their pain on a scale of 0 to 10. The scale is calibrated for each patient who is told that 0 is equal to no pain and 10 equals passing a kidney stone (male patients) or childbirth (female patients). Given the subjective nature of this scale, clinicians never perform statistical treatments of isolated reports or compare pain numbers across patients. Rather, the NPRS is used to measure pain change. So if a new narcotic is being tested on a patient population, then the clinicians are hoping that a statistically significant portion of the patient population will report a statistically significant reduction in pain. A variety of numerically based pain scales are used primarily for quick-assessment or narcotics studies. Another popular inventory is the visual analog scale (VAS), which presents the various levels of pain as a series of increasingly unhappy-looking emoticons. This is used primarily with children and the mentally disabled, and when there is a doctor-patient language barrier. Psychologists and psychiatrists have developed a number of more exhaustive pain inventories that quantify the impact on a patient's quality of life. These tests are designed to measure things like sleep disturbance, changes in diet, sexual activity, or loss of work productivity. Fundamentally, these and other pain measures are means of quantifying patient report, with most designed specifically for RCTs rather than for clinical care (an issue that will come up again later).

The Ontology That Wasn't

As figure 1.1 indicates, the biochemical and empirical-discursive are not the only pain-qua-object ontologies in contemporary biomedical discourse. The scholarly landscape of pain medicine makes regular reference to a metaphysics of pain that is psychological in nature. Indeed, the idea that there exists both physical types and psychological types of pain is a common conception of our cultural landscape. Certainly, we make somewhat routine reference to the pain of loss, the pain of sadness, and the pain of anger—the issue Morris describes as the "myth of two pains."

When it comes to pain in medical discourse, there is, indeed, a myth of two pains, but it is less about differentiating one type of pain from different from another than it is a suggestion that medical discourse actually discusses two different types of pain. In fact, within the history of medical discourse, discussions of psychological pain are largely absent. I do not object to Morris's suggestion that there are two different conceptions of pain working at cross-purposes in Western culture writ large. Indeed, there are, and they are aptly described as physical and mental. However, when analyzed within a rhetorical-ontological approach, the practices of historical psychology and psychiatry are more apt to stage a biochemical ontology onto which a study of the psychological reactions to physical pain is explored.

When Morris and others discuss psychological or mental pain, they often refer to the suffering that follows difficult or painful life events or the suffering attendant to a psychological disorder. In terms of traumatic events, scholars often discuss the types of pain that arise from heartbreak—the loss of a meaningful relationship, the failure to achieve some long-held dream, or the death of a loved one. Additionally, other scholars discuss the pain that follows witnessing or being subject to violent events—such as war or rape. Finally, there is a rich literature on comorbid pain with depression or anxiety disorders. Despite all this, the suffering that results from these various issues does not, for the medical community, result in pain. Indeed, the psychological and psychiatric community has developed its own nomenclature in order to distinguish mental suffering from pain (that is, the subjective experience of nociception). Psychologists use terms like "anxiety," "negative affect," "loss of motivation," and "depressed mood" to refer to the discomfort that arises from psychological issues. More to the point, they have held since Freud that any pain felt in such situations is most likely physical pain due to anxiety-induced muscle tension (Melzack & Wall, 1982, p. 21).

Nevertheless, there is an identifiable subdiscipline known as the "psychology of pain." Though it did not emerge until around the 1950s, this field, by and large, does not have a history of studying mental pain. Rather, pain psychologists tend to study the psychological responses to nociception—the subjective response to physical pain. The pain itself is still understood within the nociceptive metaphysics as a stimulus transmitted from a pain receptor to the brain. It is at this point—the terminus of the transmission—where psychology begins:

> Psychological and anthropological studies have shown that pain is not simply a function of the amount of bodily damage alone. Rather the amount and quality of pain we feel are also determined by our previous experiences and how well we remember them, by our ability to understand the cause of the pain and to grasp its consequences. . . . Stimuli that produce intolerable pain in one person may be tolerated without a whimper by another. . . . . Pain perception, then, cannot be defined simply in terms of particular kinds of stimuli. Rather, it is a highly personal experience, depending on cultural learning, the meaning of the situation, and other factors that are unique to each individual. (Melzack & Wall, 1982, p. 15)

Decades of study in the psychology of pain have replicated this approach. Pain psychologists have developed robust theories accounting for pain behaviors such as catastrophization—an overwhelmed response to the unfamiliar. Additionally, psychologists have charted the impact of pain on a broad array of quality-of-life issues like productivity, continence, sex drive, sleep, and so on. And while all of this research has been conducted from a largely psychological perspective, it still rests primarily on a biochemical ontology of pain.

Those familiar with the broader psychology of pain are no doubt raising some important objections: What about imagined pain? What about
psychosomatic pain? What about phantom limb? Broadly speaking, these
and many similar disorders fall under the rubric of psychogenic (formerly
psychosomatic) pain. The current vernacular suggests that psychogenic
pain might be akin to the mental and emotional pain discussed in other
arenas. I object to this suggestion for two reasons: (1) psychogenic pain
is usually understood as a phenomenon wherein psychological conditions
mimic physical pain, and (2) psychogenic pain as a concept is broadly de-
cried as a convenient label for pain not (yet) properly understood. As
Morris (1991) notes, "Traditional medicine, not surprisingly, does not
know what to do with psychogenic pain, except to deny that it exists; the
term itself is quite controversial" (p. 157). Furthermore, in addition to flat
denial, clinicians even frequently link psychogenic pain with preexisting
physiological pain. As Morris elaborates:

> Although the concept of psychogenic pain normally implies that there is no
> identifiable organic cause, two eminent doctors remind their colleagues that
> psychogenic pain commonly expresses itself as "an elaboration" of pain already
> arising from tissue damage. Perhaps an injury has healed, but the pain—for
> reasons unknown—simply refuses to stop, as if the brain had encoded it in a
> neural circuit that, once started, cannot be shut off. (p. 157)

Melzack and Wall specifically identify psychogenic pain as a diagnosis for
the otherwise undiagnosable:

> It is clear that we must recognize the psychological contribution to pain, but
> we must maintain a balanced view of it. The term "psychogenic" assumes that
> medical diagnosis is so perfect that all organic causes of pain can be detected;
> regrettably, we are far from such infallibility." (1982, p. 34)

The inclusion of this caveat in Melzack and Wall is all the more suggestive
given that they are primary proponents of a balanced view of pain that
treats physical and psychological pain equally.

When it comes to the lack of a psychological pain ontology, there is,
perhaps, one exception. Renée Leriche, considered by many to be the
first pain specialist, studied pain at the University of Strasbourg in France
from around 1910 until the 1940s. His masterwork, *The Surgery of Pain*
(1939)—an edited collection of lectures designed to be a comprehensive
study of pain from both a laboratory and a clinical perspective—is a text

uniquely out of time and would not become mainstream until the 1970s and 1980s. In Leriche's dedication to detailed investigation, he sought to elucidate and evaluate understandings of pain that come from a variety of different traditions. He devoted substantial passages to literary and philosophical conceptions of pain (pp. 24–27), but any mention of psychological pain is distinctly absent. Of course, that may be merely an oversight on Leriche's part, but I doubt it. It seems to me that if there were a then-extant psychological discourse on pain, he would have mentioned it somewhere among the laboratory, clinical, literary, and philosophical sections.

So why I am even bothering to address a metaphysics labeled "psychological pain" if it is not staged by medical practices? The answer to this question is to be found in the contemporary efforts aimed at unifying the physiological ontologies and metaphysics with the psychological alternatives. Biopsychosocial pain advocates constantly refer to a programmatic regime of engagement primarily concerned with psychological pain. Even though a detailed historical study suggests there never was such a regime, its supposed existence exerts considerable force in contemporary practice. This quasi-existence for the psychological pain ontology is why I have chosen to diagram this branch in the cladogram (fig. 1.1) in grayscale rather than black. One last point before leaving this ontology. Here is yet another moment where the affordances of an ontological history are manifest. A theoretical/metaphysical history would identify psychological pain as an equal alongside other metaphysics and subsequently focus on the Cartesian divide. Indeed, that's precisely what most histories and sociologies of pain medicine do. For example, Melzack (1973) and Melzack and Wall (1982) each include chapters on an intendant psychology of pain. Furthermore, Morris (1991), Rey (1993), and Gillian Bendelow and Simon Williams (1995) each describe a historical psychology of pain that was (or should be) integrated into a new multidisciplinary approach. However, a focus on practices and emergent ontologies highlights the fact that there really is no practical regime of engagement that stages a psychological ontology. Rather, this ontology is but a rhetorical artifact for a different purpose.

Toward Nonmodern Ontologies of Pain

Toward the end of the 1970s, four extant pain metaphysics were staged by medical practices: (1) Pain as indexical sign was alive and well in much the same way as it had been since antiquity. (2) Pain as nociception had enjoyed more than sixty years of clinical and scientific success and was easily the dominant object metaphysics. (3) Pain as statistical construct was in its infancy, but after nearly a decade of RCTs, it was coming into its own. And (4) psychological pain was a constant facet of literary and philosophical discourse and widely presumed to be undergoing continuing scrutiny within the arena of pain psychology.

The manifest multiplicities of pain helped to create an ideal environment for the inauguration of the radically new approach to pain mentioned in the introduction: the biopsychosocial/nonmodern approach. As I have been alluding to throughout this chapter, the above historical treatment was designed to provide a foundation for understanding the new pain ontologies and corresponding metaphysics that have emerged only in the past forty years and are still working at coming to prominence. These ontologies (nonmodern-practical and nonmodern-discursive) are staged in their own particular regimes of practical engagement (multimodal pain management and pain management theory, respectively) and have spawned two truly fascinating metaphysics: hybrid pain and the phenomenology of suffering. I have dubbed them "hybrid" or "nonmodern" models of pain because they are grounded (often explicitly) in a rejection of the Cartesian mind/body divide. In short, hybrid models of pain argue that pain is a phenomenon or collection of phenomena that defy the mind/body binary. Pain, under these rubrics, is always mental *and* physical, always subjective *and* objective, always hybrid. These new approaches to pain medicine often reject the historically dominant ontologies. For these reasons, hybrid and nonmodern pain ontologies represent significant breaks from mainstream medical history. However, due to the profoundly revolutionary nature of these new approaches, the rhetorical battle for acceptance and legitimacy is still ongoing.

In the chapters that follow, I will explore the efforts of new coalitions of multidisciplinary medical professions work to enact and legitimize their new pain ontologies. Additionally, I will interrogate how these new ontologies and their emergent metaphysics trouble and circulate in the material and regulatory structures that surround and penetrate the practices of pain management. But while I conclude my historical discussion of pain medicine to focus next on nonmodern pain practitioners, the contemporary state of pain science and medicine is by no means static or at an end. In fact, the chapters that follow offer a case study of continuing ontological change and multiplicity—or, in the operational metaphor of this chapter, continued evolution wherein some ontologies and the disease they enact persist and others become extinct.

CHAPTER TWO

Praxiography of Representation

In the summer of 2006, I attended my first meeting of the Midwest Pain Group (MPG). I had never been to the research site before, so I followed the directions provided to me by Google Maps (printed out on a sheet of paper, because it was 2006) until I arrived at a strip mall on the outskirts of a medium-size midwestern city. Next to an ostensibly French pizza delivery shop was a small restaurant that the MPG had rented out for the evening. A handwritten sign on the door informed me that the restaurant had been reserved for a private party, and I recognized a few of the people trickling in as belonging to the MPG, so I followed. The door opened into a bar where an MPG representative had set up a table for new members to pay and for established members to pick up their name tags—of which there was an impressive array. Nearly a hundred of the little laminated cards spread out across the table, each listing a name, highest degree earned, and medical subspecialty. There were name tags for general practitioners, nurses, chiropractors, psychologists, psychiatrists, anesthesiologists, physical therapists, pharmacists, and more. The alphabet soup that followed the names was just as varied, and included BS, BSN, MS, MSN, PhD, MD, DO, PharmD, FACS, JD, and so on. Since I'd negotiated access by offering my web design skills, I was provided membership in the MPG and a name tag that read "Scott Graham, MS/ Webmaster." (Of course, I had an MA, not an MS, but I decided not to mention it.)

Past the bar and around the corner from the extensive wine rack, ten long rectangular tables had been set in rows in the main dining area. All were oriented toward a wall with a white screen illuminated by an LCD projector, depicting a sketch of a man in a black suit with devil horns sitting on a throne of skulls overlooking the fires of hell and a simple caption:

"HMO Claims Adjustor." (I later learned that the president of the MPG tried to find a new insurance industry cartoon for each monthly meeting.) At this point, the room was about half full. Doctors, nurses, chiropractors, psychologists, attorneys, and pharmaceutical representatives were ordering drinks, finding seats, talking to friends, and comparing case notes. In short, the dining room was filled with the dull hum of polite conversation.

As more members arrived, the hum escalated to a roar until the agreed-upon start time when the MPG president tapped his microphone to get the crowd's attention and switched the projector to the first of four Power-Point presentations for the evening. The president—a doctor of osteopathy who specializes in pain medicine—introduced the first presenter, a pharmaceutical representative from Endo. A lively and engaging speaker, she addressed the crowd on the benefits and proper usage of the fentanyl patch. Fentanyl is a schedule 2 narcotic, which means it's a prescription opioid, and it is commonly used for chronic pain. The patch, as the name suggests, is a topical delivery system—that is, it attaches to the patient's skin (much like a nicotine patch) and delivers a time-release dose of fentanyl directly to the pained area. The drug rep spoke for about ten minutes, referring regularly to the PowerPoint slides, which had clearly been designed by a professional graphic artist. The slides juxtaposed anguished faces with relieved faces, bar charts with scatter plots, and clinical data with blatant advertisement. When the presentation was over, the time for questions and answers began.

This is when the real work of the MPG started. FDA regulations and pharmaceutical business practices require that during a presentation, a pharmaceutical representative can only talk about the proven and approved uses. In short, they must confine themselves to discussing only those doses, applications, and uses approved and indicated by the FDA. However, when it comes to question-and-answer time at the MPG, all bets are off. The MPG members questioned the representative about study limitations, potential uses outside the FDA indication, specific cases they had experienced in which the patch did not perform as they'd anticipated, and ways to use the patch in combination with other therapies. But the membership did not only address Endo's representative. The entire conversation sparked lively debate among MPG members, generating discussion across disciplinary boundaries and levels of education.

As debate continued, a real point of contention arose. Apparently, patients using the patch for the first time reported that they experienced a cool, tingling sensation. No one knew why, but as good scientifically minded practitioners, the MPG members wanted answers. Why would it tingle? Was it the fentanyl? Was it the patch glue? Was it the combination? The Endo representative didn't know. A physiologist's and a pharmacist's speculations contradicted each other. And then, the drug rep remembered that the Endo gift bag everyone had been graciously provided included a placebo patch as a sample. The room paused for a moment, and then, en masse, dove into their swag bags, used the free Endo scissors to open the free Endo placebo, and began sticking—to themselves—the sample patch. The room was alight with discovery as member after member exclaimed, "It does tingle! It must be the glue!"

Though the identification of the tingling agent in the fentanyl patch is likely not the most important discovery ever made at an MPG meeting, this vignette does, indeed, describe my first encounter with the group, and perfectly captures its members' spirit of engagement and collaboration. In observed settings and follow-up interviews, the MPG members repeatedly shared their passionate investment in reducing pain and improving health. They also reported that the MPG had been instrumental in their efforts to do just that. But that combination of passion, commitment, and past success does not mean their efforts have been easy or even entirely successful. Indeed, the MPG members confront myriad challenges in attempting to establish and refine a nonmodern pain ontology. The longstanding dominance of the semiotic and biochemical pain ontologies are only two such difficulties. Integrating practices from the MPG's twenty-plus different subspecialties would constitute an impressive feat of cross-ontological calibration. Members from different regimes of practice not only come to the MPG participating in different pain ontologies, they also have fundamentally different approaches concerning the metaphysics of the human body, the ontology of disease, and the proper epistemology for health and/or medical science. These fundamental differences in practice and theory make it difficult (but not impossible, as the incommensurability thesis predicts) for MPG members to embrace research and practice from disciplines whose basic concepts do not match those of their own.

Nevertheless the MPG as an organization and the members as individuals are strongly committed to establishing a new approach both to pain science and medicine. They seek a new ontology that integrates both the insights from prior ontologies as well as the myriad number of regimes of practice in pain management. They hope to foster a new form of medical practice that utilizes therapies and interventions from a wide variety of regimes to pursue new—sometimes grander—goals for health care.

The MPG actively pursues these goals despite the many challenges from traditional disciplinary medicine, preestablished ontologies, and political-economic forces. It is these efforts by the MPG that serve as the primary focus of the next two chapters. More specifically, in this chapter, I explore how to provide an account of a setting like the MPG using a hybrid rhetorical-ontological approach. How to do so is a more fraught question than it might initially seem. As I describe below, a rhetorical-ontological investigation of a deliberative space, like the MPG, runs contrary to a major thrust in new materialisms that rejects all inquiry into representation. And, of course, inquiry into representation is the foundation of rhetorical studies. This conflict between rhetorical studies and anti-representationalist strains of new materialisms makes a hybrid rhetorical-ontological approach quite difficult. Making a space for something like traditional rhetorical inquiry without sliding backward into (post-)modernism presents a significant obstacle.

Subsequently, this chapter offers a detailed description of the practice of the MPG—the practical activity that occurs within an ostensibly "deliberative" space. Using this description as a foundation, I argue for what I dub a "praxiography of representation" focused on the practices of "cross-ontological calibration." As the name suggests, a praxiography of representation focuses not so much on what people say or what texts mean but rather on how representational activity circulates within and contributes to a deeper ecology of practices in which those acts of representation are embedded. Cross-ontological calibration is one form of representational practice that serves to navigate the boundaries among divergent ontologies. Ontological calibration is at the core of what the MPG does. And as I argue below, it is the place where the anti-representationalist strains of new materialisms leave off and where rhetorical-ontological inquiry truly begins.

A New Ontology and MPG Practice

In chapter 1, I began to explore the broader exigencies that led to the establishment of organizations like the MPG. The four long-standing pain ontologies and their particular histories are active participants in the reality that MPG members face. As such, I will now explore the MPG where I left off in the previous chapter—with the origins of the fifth and sixth pain ontologies in the early 1970s. While the objectification and subsequent medicalization of pain began as early as the advent of modernity, medical science of the 1970s took the discourse of pain to a previously unreached level of complexity. The 1970s marked the rise of the International Association for the Study of Pain (IASP), the first major professional body with pain as its primary object of knowledge. The founding of this *multidisciplinary*[1] body of health-care providers and researchers ushered in a new era of pain inquiry and pain management health care. Capitalizing on the research of previous eras, the IASP and its affiliates pursued a broad research agenda designed to unify the preexisting pain ontologies. Indeed, the researchers of this era vigorously investigated pain as nociception, psychological pain, and pain as statistical construct—all research agendas still active today.

These clinicians and scientists invented instruments like the numeric pain rating scale (NPRS) and the visual analog scale (VAS), discussed in the last chapter. The now widely used McGill pain questionnaire defines a list of acceptable adjectives for describing pain—for example, *tugging, burning, splitting, nagging,* and *dreadful* (Melzack, 1973). They divided pain into identifiable subtypes: somatic, neuropathic, and psychogenic. They developed statistical methods for quantifying the impact of pain on the patient's quality of life, psychological well-being, and economic livelihood. Additionally, this flurry of research into the nature and treatments of pain fostered the development of multiple agencies that regulate and certify practitioners' qualification to practice pain management (the IASP, the American Pain Foundation, the American Board of Pain Medicine, the American Pain Society and the American Academy for Pain Management). Fellowships, internships, and student clinical rotations are now common in pain medicine. A number of disciplinary journals are devoted exclusively to the study and treatment of pain, including *Pain, Pain Practice, Pain Medicine, Pain Physician,* and *Journal of Pain.* In short, the study of pain is now a full-fledged science, and the practice of pain management health care has become its own amalgam of technoscientific organizations and practices.

Foundational to this new engagement with pain was, and still is, the attempt to establish a nonmodern ontology, which would only be made possible by the establishment of a new hybrid model for health in general: the biopsychosocial model, pioneered by George Engel and presented to the broader medical community in a 1977 article in *Science.* In "The Need for a New Medical Model: A Challenge for Biomedicine," Engel objects to the reductive biomedical model of disease that was then (and to a certain extent still is) ubiquitous across health disciplines. As an alternative, he suggested an approach grounded in systems modeling that treats biological, social, and psychological factors as coequals in an interactional matrix of causality for disease. Engel cautions against treating the physical body separately from the mind and recommended instead that health care should recognize "the psychobiological unity of man" (p. 133). Though this new model certainly has not become uniform across the medical disciplines, it is nearly ubiquitous in contemporary psychology and also serves as a foundational construct for efforts to establish a new pain ontology.

Amid these ongoing international efforts to establish a new pain ontology, the MPG became active in 2004 and was, in its infancy, a very informal organization. For years, its founder—Dr. Peters, a doctor of osteopathic medicine (DO) with five board certifications[2] (two in pain medicine, one in headache medicine, one in internal medicine, and one in hospice care)—had been working through the difficulties of pain medicine alone in his private practice. Through a combination of his education in pain science and medicine and his experience as a clinician, he began to recognize the need for a multidisciplinary approach to pain (Peters, ethnographic interview). So Peters invited a few of his close colleagues in his referral network—another pain physician, a couple of psychologists, and a pharmacist—to start meeting on a semi-regular basis to talk about the latest innovations in pain medicine. Thus, an informal pain reading group was formed.

In this early stage of the proto-MPG, Peters and the other members would share recent journal articles on new theories about and approaches to pain management. Their primary goal was self-education. They would read the articles, meet, and discuss the possible uses and/or limitations of each study. This focus on education and scholarly research (and implicitly EBM), which can be traced back to the founding of the group, continues today. Indeed, the current incarnation of the MPG mission statement reflects these goals:

> The [Midwest Pain Group] is devoted to education and research in pain management. We are a multidisciplinary nonprofit professional organization and feel it is critical to maintain a variety of represented health care professionals within our group. We are not a restricted organization and are open to any health care professional interested in pain and its management.

At the time of my study (2006–2009), the MPG was still primarily a journal club; however, its expanding membership had required changes in venue and format. The setting and format of MPG meetings are aptly described by the vignette at the beginning of this chapter.[3] During my study, it was not atypical for seventy to eighty practitioners from more than twenty different disciplines and subspecialties (including acupuncture, anesthesiology, alternative medicine, chiropractic medicine, family medicine, gerontology, internal medicine, law, nursing, orthopedics, osteopathy, pain medicine, pharmacology, pharmacy, physiatry, physical therapy, physiology, psychiatry, psychology, and surgery) to attend the meetings, held the third Wednesday of each month. The opening vignette, while typical of the format and engagement of MPG members, is not, however, representative of a meeting's usual content. Though the MPG was often sponsored (at least in part) by pharmaceutical corporations, those companies seldom provided speakers.

In fact, the vast majority of the presentations were offered by MPG members, frequently criticized the research supporting the sponsoring pharmaceutical organization—one reason why the MPG was often short on funding. Using a combination of membership dues, educational grants, and pharmaceutical funding, MPG meetings provided members with meals, drinks, and photocopies of relevant articles and PowerPoint presentations. Typically, drug or medical technology companies would choose to sponsor a particular MPG meeting. While this sponsorship determined the theme of the evening, it typically did not determine the nature of the discussion—the majority of MPG meeting discussions were usually balanced in their support and criticism of the sponsoring organization's product. Meeting themes typically revolved around either an ailment or an intervention. For example, I attended meetings on illnesses such as osteoarthritis of the knee, migraines, fibromyalgia, postherpetic neuralgia, and failed back surgery syndrome. Additionally, I observed programs devoted to interventions such as acupuncture, spinal cord stimulation, pregabalin therapy, physiotherapy, cognitive-behavioral therapy, and Synvisc injections. Since the open-ended discussion model that served the group in its infancy would be logistically impossible for the MPG's expanded size, the organization developed its own suite of presentation genres—adapted from common genres and health care and education more broadly. These presentations served as the foundation of discussion as much as the research on which they were based. I have labeled these dominant presentation genres—which developed organically and informally—article summary, article synthesis, basic science presentation, and practice reflection. Each followed a specific format and convention and generally evoked the same type, quality, and duration of conversation.

The *article summaries*—much as the name suggests—were straight-forward recapitulations of a selected clinical study. Generally, these were studies of clinical efficacy trials from a wide range of journals, including (but not limited to) *Neuroscience, Journal of Pain Symptom Management, Pain, Archives of Physical Medicine/Rehabilitation, Headache, Cephalgia,* the *Clinical Journal of Pain, Pain Medicine,* and the *Journal of Opioid Management.* The accompanying presentation and PowerPoint slides usually followed the research article's format, with generic slots for intro-duction, background, subject selection, study methods, results, discussion, limitations, and conclusions. Typically, the presenter would highlight ad-ditional study limitations not raised by the author(s). Most MPG meet-ings began with a prominent efficacy trial for a pain management drug or procedure promoted by the evening's sponsor—most often a drug com-pany. This material exigency was no doubt one of the primary reasons for the dominance of this genre. It was not uncommon for article summaries to be assigned to students on clinical rotations with MPG members. The following excerpt from a pharmacy student's article summary on the use of pregabalin for cases of central neuropathic pain associated with spinal cord injury is quite typical:

> My article is "Pregabalin in Central Neuropathic Pain Associated with Spinal Cord Injury." The International Association for the Study of Pain defines cen-tral pain as pain caused by lesion or a dysfunction in the CNS, so situations such as spinal cord injury, stroke, multiple sclerosis, or amyoplasia can cause central neuropathic pain. About 40 percent of patients with spinal injury have central neuropathic pain, and that is the type of pain that will be the focus of today's study. The objective of the study is to evaluate how effective it is for Lyrica [pre-gabalin] to work in central neuropathic pain, and the central neuropathic pain for this one is associated with spinal cord injury only. The duration of the study was 12 weeks long, and all the patient was randomized and the patient was— all the data was collected from a multicenter pain clinic in Australia. All the analyses were based on the intent to treat, so all the patients, even those who [dropped] out, were included in the study. In order to be included in the study, you had to have at least one dose of medication or have at least one baseline assessment. (MPG Journal Club, March 2007)

As you can see, the article summary genre generally follows the conven-tions of a conference presentation, except that the MPG presenter seldom actually conducted the study. He or she simply reported the study's ratio-nale, methods, results, and limitations.

Article syntheses were much like truncated oral versions of review articles. A member of the MPG would select approximately three to six recent articles on a topic related to the meeting's theme. The selected articles could be from a single discipline (such as orthopedic surgery in the case of one presentation on chronic low-back pain) or intensely multidisciplinary. Article syntheses often arose out of presenter dissatisfaction with an article selected (or assigned) for a summary presentation. A common invocation to an article synthesis would begin with a statement like this one from a February 2007 meeting on postconcussive syndrome:

> [Dr. Peters] asked me to speak tonight about the use of dihydroergotamine in patients with postconcussive syndrome. It's an article that was actually published in the journal *Headache* in 1994. I was a little surprised that he had asked me to present a journal article that was so old. . . . I spent some time reading the article and then I did a literature search this afternoon to see if there were more recent studies so I could give you guys some comparative and contrastive. (MPG Journal Club, February 2007)

Article syntheses then were often driven by clarifying or improving upon a primary article under discussion. In the following extract from an earlier presentation in the same meeting, the presenter provides what she believes to be essential background information for understanding the current study at issue.

> These two studies had more to do with how many patients had migraine and how many patients were diagnosed with migraine correctly according to the International Headache Society criteria, the latest version of which is now 2004, so the criteria have changed a little bit. Basically, at that time in 1989, about 38 percent of those who should achieve a diagnosis had achieved a diagnosis, and about 62 percent had not. By 1999—and remember, this is post, now, Imitrex, Maxalt, Zomig—all those triptans have been released. We've long since had Depakote approved by the FDA for migraine prevention. Most docs knew about topiramate who were doing a lot of migraine already. Despite that, we're still only getting about 48 percent diagnosed. Well, unfortunately, now we're gonna pull ahead to 2007—at least that's the publication date of this article—and we're about in the same boat. Now, this article goes a step further to say, "Well, OK, that's very interesting they're diagnosed, but which of them are treated prophylactically with some type of preventive medication if they should be?" They found that about 32, roughly—you can quibble about point percentages—but around 32 to 33 percent had severe migraine by criteria of the amount of dis-

ability, in particular, that were not being treated with preventive therapy. Now, about 13 percent were not being treated who had mild or mild-to-moderate disease. The total number is about 38 percent weren't being treated who probably should have been. (MPG Journal Club, February 2007)

Basic science presentations were probably the only ones explicitly recognized as a genre by members of the MPG. These presentations—typically delivered by a physiologist or a neuroscientist—aimed to inform members about the nature and cause(s) of a given ailment. Adopting the standard nomenclature of Western biomedicine, these generally very biomechanistic presentations typically explained the "etiology" and "pathogenesis" of the chosen disorder. Etiology and pathogenesis are the subfields of medical science devoted to identifying the specific cause(s) and clinical progression of diseases. Below is a typical example from physiologist Dr. Fitzpatrick on the neurophysiology of addiction:

There's a lot of interesting things going on with addiction and our understanding of the underpinnings of what is going on. There's some really interesting things that occur physiologically with what is going on in addiction in terms of substance abuse, but also in terms of behaviors. What we're finding is that they're one and the same. . . .

Let's look at these and look at some of the nervous system aspects here [on key areas on a map of the brain]. First let's look at that reward pathway. Kinda the down and dirty of it, if you will. This is that reward circuit. The prefrontal/frontal cortex. This is the decision area. This is executive function. I always tell the students, this is where your mother resides. This is where your control over your behaviors—you decide to say something. Your mother taught you, if you can't say something nice, don't say anything, right? If I asked you what you thought of my tie and you're sitting there thinking, "He paid money for that?" OK. He's not gonna say that 'cause he doesn't wanna hurt my feelings. He has some empathy for me because he's got some ties sorta like that at home as well. He'll say, "It's different." That's that prefrontal cortex. It has a big control on decision making, on the control of those behaviors. Medial dorsal thalamus—the thalamus is always a gateway to the cortex, so you're tying in anything that goes up to the cortex has to come through the thalamus. You always have to have a thalamic nuclei tied into anything. (MPG Journal Club, January 2006)

Finally, *practice reflections* articulated recent research with the clinical practice of the presenter. Practice reflections were a variable genre and often took several different forms, most commonly the case study. These presentations explored the successes and failures involved in treating a particular patient. Case studies explicitly recognize that the subject selection criteria of clinical trials are designed to eliminate variables and thus elides the complexity of many patients. Pain patients, in particular, typically have complicated case histories and a variety of comorbid conditions that complicate treatment. Exploring the nuances of one specific patient allowed MPG members to reflect on the articulations between the ideals of academic research and the reality of clinical practice. The other common variant of the practice reflection is a hybrid genre that unifies conventions from both the article-based presentations and the case study. This variant usually followed the format of an article summary or synthesis but with frequent pauses for the presenter to reflect on a particular patient's history that was relevant to the issue at hand.[4] This variant is exemplified in the following passage presented by an interventional anesthesiologist at a 2006 MPG meeting:

> I work in the pain clinic and I see patients. I'm an interventional anesthesiologist, so I do a lot of blocks. . . . I'm not as bad as the dentists, but I put needles into people, and that hurts, but some pain for some gain. What I'm gonna talk about is whiplash injury, and that brings to the zygapophyseal joint pain, or the facet joint pains. That's funny because I have, I would say, 5 percent of my patients, or 1, 2 percent may have some fibromyalgia. Some of those patients—as we have a clinic diagnosis, just as a clinical diagnosis by the American College of Rheumatologists—those patients, they have other painful syndromes as well. A lot of those patients, they have some osteoarthritis of the spine, and sometimes, they have this referred facet joint pain from the neck or from the lumbar spine. I can tell you I probably have more than ten patients who came just for fibromyalgia diagnosis and they start to examine the patients, did an MRI, no radiculopathy, but have neck pains, pains in the trapezius muscle, paraspinous muscle, and other points as well. They also had, on top of the fibromyalgia, neck pain coming from the facet joints at the cervical level and the lumbar level. (MPG Journal Club, February 2006)

Every presentation, regardless of genre, was designed to initiate conversation among the membership. (Of course, success in generating discussion often varies according to genre, presentation content, and presenter style.) The discussions following article summaries and syntheses often revolved around study limitations—both in design and statistical reliability. Questions following basic science presentations were often solely clarifying in nature. However, the discussions following practice reflections were often quite engaged, with explanations of the supporting or dissenting case and debate over clinical applicability. The discussions following each genre are the points at which members shared information across disciplinary specialties and, thus, at which the group confronted the differences between disciplinary languages and research traditions. In these post-presentation discussions, members frequently talked "off-label," discussing treatments, theories, and practice that violate the tight regulations imposed by disciplines, regulatory agencies, and insurance company policies.

Talking "Off-Label"

Talking "off-label" was the metaphor one of the group members coined to defer certain questions to the "unofficial" discussion following his presentation of data from clinical trials. Talking off-label also became a metaphor for the larger efforts of the MPG to overcome the reductive vocabularies and limited treatments of pain that follow from narrow disciplinarily and regulatory restrictions. The label on a prescription drug, especially the schedule 2 opiates that are often prescribed for severe pain, is a highly specific product of scientific trials, legal disclaimers and responsibilities, and regulatory approval processes. The drug label compresses an enormous amount of scientific, legal, and regulatory discourse into a localized and binding statement. MPG members had to talk off-label in a variety of ways to accomplish their goals and to navigate restrictions on the dialogue between research and clinical practice. They needed to discuss pain as understood outside their disciplines, treatment interventions not common to their fields, and research from different ontologies. When they explored unsanctioned indications of approved treatments, the MPG members stepped outside their disciplinary restrictions and those of the medical-industrial complex and attempted to foster a better understanding of pain science, thereby improving the multidisciplinary, cross-ontological practices of pain management.

The following excerpt from a 2006 MPG presentation on the role of cognitive-behavioral therapy in preparing patients for spinal cord stimulation offers a good example of an off-label discussion. Spinal cord stimulators are fascinating cyborg-esque computer devices surgically implanted in patients who suffer from chronic low-back pain. A series of electrodes threaded into the spinal column deliver constant, low-intensity electrical stimulation, which essentially overloads pain processing in the brain and prevents the transmission of pain stimuli. Despite the very biomechanical-sounding nature of this intervention, it was actually made possible by Melzack's (1973) work on a nonmodern—or, in his parlance, "gate-control"—theory of pain. The biopsychosocial focus on pain processing encouraged pain researchers to think in new ways about pain processing as opposed to mere transmission. And many pain management specialists who install spinal cord stimulators recognize that psychological evaluations and treatment are an important antecedent to surgery. Simultaneous depression, for example, can limit the effectiveness of spinal cord stimulation. In the following excerpt, pain management specialist Dr. Peters works with psychologist Dr. Green to highlight these biopsychosocial interrelations for the broader MPG audience.

DR. GREEN: We got her depression under control. . . . She has a very intrusive mother, and there were problems with the intrusive mother we dealt with. Kind of an absent father. A bunch of other family issues we dealt with that helped her get her depression under control, as well as the medication changes.

DR. PETERS: You have data? You said there was an article about improvements in outcomes with psychological treatment versus no treatment versus interventional. Is that true?

DR. GREEN: I have a whole stack of research when I first started doing spinal cord stimulator evaluations that demonstrate that there's a significant group of patients who look like they will benefit, but if they have significant depression, you can . . . think things are wonderful, do the implant, and within a few months, they're not benefiting. If you treat their depression, they appear to be able to have the procedure, to benefit from it, and have a long-term benefit.

DR. PETERS: One more question. Don't you think that would also relate to any other kinds of treatment besides the spinal cord stimulator, like medications, physical therapy? Wouldn't that—just from a theoretical perspective now—wouldn't it predispose that we're not gonna do as well with medical therapy, with[out] other interventions?

DR. GREEN: I'd certainly like to believe that. That's what my whole practice is built around, Jim. [*Laughter.*]

DR. PETERS: I was giving you a lead-in there, Simon.

DR. GREEN: Yeah. If you don't deal with psychological issues, your probability for outcome is gonna be less. If you've got a pain disorder and there's any muscle input, any kind of elevated anxiety, anxiety issues, it is gonna affect resting muscle tension and your ability to be effective there. If someone's depressed, you have such great perceptual biases with depression, I think sometimes they can be better and not even have enough disruption of concentration, attention, et cetera, and be kind of a gray-lens focus that they didn't even see the improvements. I think that's part of what you do in psychotherapy with pain patients—is you help them identify improvements. A lot of psychotherapy's about inspiring hope, and talk about a group that, when they get to me, is usually pretty low in hope, so help them identify positives that they just can't see in these situations. (MPG Journal Club, January 2006)

I reprint this extended passage here because it is an exemplar of the off-label discussion that is the cornerstone of my exploration of the MPG. And it's important to note that I'm not the only person to identify this off-label discourse as so essential to the work of the MPG and the clinical practice it informs. Over and over again, interview subjects identified how much more productive their work seemed to be when the presentations often promoted engaged cross-ontological debate and conversation— that is, off-label discourse. For example, psychologist Dr. Freedman, when asked which presentations were the most helpful, responded:

We have a variety of different presentation formats which are useful in their own ways. I guess some of the ones I found the most helpful are when somebody presents basic information, and we use it as a jumping-off point. So that's created the most discussion. I like that. And from time to time, I think it's also good when you have the presentations that are very didactic. . . . I think where it gets most fun is when you cut into the talks, whether it's presenting an article or a topic you present something and you really open it up for discussion, and that seems to really get a lot of people going. (Freedman, ethnographic interview)

Similarly, Dr. Boysen extolled the virtues of off-label discourse in the wake of presentations over methodologically weak articles:

I think what was useful was not some of the—I have to put this in quotes— "scientific" papers were less than well done. It was useful to discuss them, but I think some of the discussions about the approach to certain difficult pain problems was useful. There isn't necessarily a standard way that you can get results. I think getting feedback from a variety of different providers there was quite useful. (Boysen, ethnographic interview)

Reinforcing this theme, Dr. Bennetti reported that the off-label discussion with its engagement from multiple disciplinary perspectives is one of the most effective means at working toward a nonmodern—or, in his jargon, "mosaic"—understanding of pain: "When you sit in a group like that and start to put all the pieces of the mosaic together, you start to see the whole picture. The impact on the psychology, the basic science, the attorneys that deal with patients caught in a vortex of [legal and disability issues]" (Bennetti, ethnographic interview).

In another interview, a pharmacist, Dr. Benedict, told me that the MPG was much more helpful and successful than other organizations of which he was a member precisely because of the off-label format:

> I think the format—the Q&A—the openness lends to that. And its practitioners. The diversity of the group we have—of all the health-care professionals—that lends to the success of it. Example, our last meeting the pragmatic trials versus stage three trials/phase three trials. Pragmatic ones are really applied to practice settings rather than textbook science settings. We have practitioners in the audience, academicians, nurses, pharmacists, physical therapists—all have questions and everybody gets to ask how it affects or what it means for me and my practice area. Everybody hears that and learns from it. That's probably the most beneficial or successful. (Benedict, ethnographic interview)

Here, Dr. Benedict links two important issues for cross-disciplinary collaboration: the off-label discussion and a pragmatic orientation. Again, the shared commitment to improving patient care resulted in presentations that highlighted pragmatic issues and were more interesting and engaging, and, in Dr. Benedict's estimation, more successful. Indeed, all this feedback makes a great deal of sense given the goals of fostering cross-ontological dialogue.

One question that remains, however, is how to address and account for the role of off-label, cross-ontological dialogue within a rhetorical-ontological idiom. Typically, when it comes to cross-disciplinary dialogue, notions of incommensurability rise to the fore. However, as the previous chapter notes, the incommensurability thesis predicts irreconcilable cross-disciplinary conflict among this diverse range of discussants. At least in the case of the MPG, that conflict is manifestly not the case. The collected recordings of the MPG demonstrate that discussions like this one are routine. A great deal of effort is devoted to refining the emergent nonmodern pain ontology and articulating the new multidisciplinary practice that stages the new pain ontology and is authorized by it. Furthermore, both the demands of new materialism and the iterative relationships among MPG member discussion and practice demand an approach to these dialogues that does not construe them as isolated or solely discursive. Developing an apparatus to explore passages like the one above is, therefore, at the heart of *The Politics of Pain Medicine*. Indeed, this is precisely what I mean when I aim toward a rhetorical-ontological inquiry.

Praxiography of Representation

Rhetorical studies, of course, would have a lot to say about the discourse of the MPG. It has much to offer in terms of modes of deliberation and the relationship among those modes and biomechanical theories and clinical practices. However, a rhetorical approach would appear, at first blush, to be directly contrary to the insights of new materialisms. Rhetorical analysis traditionally comes with an attendant focus on language and representation. However, a great deal of work in new materialisms explicitly rejects inquiry into representation as in any way appropriate or desirable. For example, Coole and Frost (2010) write:

> We interpret [the move to new materialisms] as signs that the more textual approaches associated with the so-called cultural turn are increasingly being deemed inadequate for understanding contemporary society, particularly in light of some of its most urgent challenges regarding environmental, demographic, geopolitical, and economic change. (p. 3)

Similarly, Pickering (2010) understands the move toward ontological inquiry as a move away from the postmodern epistemological theories "associated with the so-called linguistic turn in the humanities and social sciences, a dualist insistence that while we have access to our own words, language, and representations, we have no access to things in themselves" (p. 26). Notably, these rejections of inquiry into representation are among the most innocuous.

While I greatly appreciate Levi Bryant's *Democracy of Objects* (2011) for its identification of the epistemic and hegemonic fallacies, it offers a deeply disturbing model of communication that serves to simultaneously enfranchise both the transmission model (à la Shannon and Weaver, 1949) and radical cosmic incommensurability. As Bryant describes it:

> Information is non-linear and system specific, existing only for the system in question and as a function of the organization or endo-structure of the object. In saying that information is non-linear, my point is that it is an effect of the endo-structure of the object as it relates to its environment and how the endo-structure resonates within the field of differential relations that define that structure. Information is not in the environment, but a product of the system perturbed by its environment. (p. 166)

Thus under Bryant's model, communication is an event wherein one object that happens to have the requisite physical features perturbs its environment (presumably by using vocal cords to vibrate the air) and a second object with the appropriate and complementary physical structures (ears) receives this annoying stimuli; due to the accidents of the second object's internal makeup (brain, linguistic training), the perturbation is interpreted as information. To elucidate this model of communication, Bryant relates a cynical narrative of how he interacts with his cat, pointing out that where he interprets the cat's nuzzles as affection, it's very likely merely a desire for warmth. The cat has perturbed (nuzzled) Bryant, and his human inculcation has interpreted that as information (affection) in a way that has nothing whatsoever to do with the cat.

And although he spends more time discussing communication with rocks and cats, Bryant claims the same model applies equally to humans communicating with humans:

> This sort of selectivity is true not only of relations with objects between different sorts, but also of relations between objects of the same sort. Many, I'm sure, have experienced and been baffled by conversations with others from very different theoretical backgrounds and orientations. In such discussions, points and claims you take for granted as obvious seem not even to be registered or noticed by the interlocutor when made. Here we have different forms of selective openness among humans in discourse. (2011, p. 174)

This presents a tremendously limited view of rhetoric and communication. Essentially, Bryant's model offers a form of hyper-incommensurability where communication as we know it is impossible—and insofar as it is possible, is merely the lucky accident of a well-timed perturbation landing on an object with an appropriate set of structures. Ultimately, this version of new materialism presents an ontology of consciousness grounded in isolated, individual, and idiosyncratic perceptions of a stable reality, perceptions that cannot be meaningfully communicated among interlocutors. As such, a rhetorical theory grounded in this form of new materialism cannot move one iota beyond the ludic postmodernism that new materialisms reject.

This hostility toward inquiry into representation and communication can make new materialisms very foreign to rhetoricians. Nevertheless, I believe that the new materialist rejection of the two-world problem is compelling enough to warrant a reinterpretation of rhetorical inquiry. The question that remains is how to do this without entirely casting off all inquiry into language. Once again, I think the solution lies in Mol's (1999, 2002) particular brand of new materialisms. However, the move to a rhetorically oriented form of ontological inquiry will require further accommodations of Mol's work. In new materialist inquiry, science and medicine are not about seeing and knowing, but rather about doing and being. For Mol, specifically, disease is done/enacted/lived differently in different spaces. In each space, the ontology of disease is different. Methodologically, multiple ontologies requires a primary focus on practices. Indeed, Mol dubs her approach a "praxiography of disease" (p. 31). Praxiography, as the name suggests, comprises a variety of ethnographic methodologies and focuses on the study of practices as opposed to the study of cultures. Praxiography moves beyond the plurality of perspectivalism into multiplicity. For Mol, there is not one atherosclerosis; there are atheroscleroses. Each site of practice—the surgery ward, the physical therapy clinic, and the pathology lab—stages its own disease ontology, its own atherosclerosis, and, in my study, its own pain.

Mol's decision to conduct her investigation in the clinical and laboratory sites of a hospital has helped her to develop an approach to multiple ontologies based on what I argue is a limited understanding of the practices of biomedicine. She does not study the clinical library, hospital administration, consultation meetings, or records and billing. Each of these nonclinical sites contributes equally to the broad mix of regimes of practical engagement that make up contemporary biomedical practices. Equally important are spaces of education and policy. In fact, such sites are essential locations for the practices of "ontological calibration" (explained in detail below) invoked, but mostly unexplored, in Mol's analysis. As such, some adaptation of multiple-ontologies analysis is required to adequately interrogate educational and policy settings. Under a strict praxiographic approach, the practices of such fora are presentational dialogue, question-and-answer periods, slideware management, and so on.

However, a sole focus on those practices and the ontologies they stage would elide the more important role of educational and policy forums to adjudicate and coordinate conflicting ontologies of pain and disease as well as the impacts those efforts have on clinical practices.

The obvious challenge, however, is that medical educators and policy discussants rarely speak in terms of practical regimes of engagement, and they almost never speak in terms of multiple ontologies. Indeed, as much of health policy is dominated by EBM and clinical research, the discourse of these spaces enacts the perspectival/representational epistemological/metaphysical orientation that multiple ontologies seek to avoid. That is, EBM is a scholarly and scientific practice. It stages an empirical-discursive ontology in that it is composed of looking (at data) and redescribing those observations (publication). But praxiographic analysts should not feel obligated to offer an explanation solely in terms that are meaningful to the participants. Ethnographers commonly make a distinction between emic and etic accounts. Emic accounts use terms meaningful to the subjects of the ethnography, whereas etic descriptions deploy terms meaningful to the ethnographer. So just as an anthropologist might describe an indigenous ritual in terms of its sociocultural (rather than spiritual) meaning, my focus will be on an ontological (rather than metaphysical/epistemological) account of the MPG, AAPM, and FDA. Following this logic, my analysis treats the stated epistemologies and metaphysics of the discussants as emergent epiphenomena that arise from their ontologies. In other words, just as certain practices stage certain ontologies, the discursive instantiation of those ontologies (as beholden to 2,500 years of epistemological/metaphysical inquiry) will necessarily be cast as perspectival and representationalist. Practices stage modes of being that in turn encourage the participants to talk about truth and knowledge in ways that are operationalized by the underlying ontology.

Put another way, my analysis will accept the new materialist move away from representation—insofar as representation is understood as correspondence epistemology. However, unwilling to throw the baby out with the bathwater, as it were, I offer a praxiography of representational practices, or praxiography of representation, as a viable alternative. As previously stated, new materialist and multiple ontological analysis is about doing. As rhetoricians are all too aware, language is doing. It has impacts and consequence—social, political, material. Rehabilitating Foucault for a project akin to new materialisms, Law (1994) offers perhaps a clearer account of this mode of inquiry (an account also cited by Mol, 2002):

My proposal is that we take the notion of discourse and cut it down to size. This means first, we should treat it as a set of patterns that might be imputed to the networks of the social; second, we should look for discourses in the plural, not discourse in the singular; third, we should treat discourses as ordering attempts, not orders; fourth, we should explore how they are performed, embodied and told in different materials; and fifth, we should consider the ways in which they interact, change, or indeed face extinction. (Law, 1994, p. 95)

Following Law, the praxiography of representation I offer will endeavor to account for the effects, rather than the hermeneutics, of representation. What representational tactics are deployed in educational and policy spaces? What are the consequences of those strategies? How do such rhetorical *technē* leverage or undercut modes of power and coordinate with materiality? How are they inhibited by structure, power, and habit?

Ontological Calibration

As I suggested above, one primary locus of inquiry for *The Politics of Pain Medicine* is sites of ontological calibration. Although disease—atherosclerosis for Mol, pain for me—is multiple, it does not have to be fractured. In keeping with her focus on specific hospital localities and the micropractices that exist there, Mol offers a vision of ontological calibration thoroughly steeped in clinical practices. Accordingly, much of the work of ontological calibration in Mol's study occurs as a patient is shuffled from wing to wing of the hospital while different, often conflicting, diagnostic data points pile up. For example, in the following passage, Mol documents the calibration exigencies that arise when subjective patient reports elicited in the diagnostic interview do not align with clinical tests aimed at evaluating vein pressure:

When the patient's feelings and the results of the pressure measurements contradict each other, they are no longer signs of a single object. The story that relates pain and pressure falters. What to do? At this point it is possible to sustain the singularity of the object, but then one signifier must be discarded. Both patient and technician make an attempt in that direction. Mr. Somers wonders whether there may be something wrong with the measurements, for he's convinced of the reality of his pain. The technician sides with "her" pressures: she downgrades Mr. Somers' feelings to "what all you feel" and gladly shifts the responsibility of dealing with these findings further back to the doctor. What is this doctor to do? Two diverging signs cannot have a single object as their common source. But on the form the patient carries from the vascular laboratory back to the outpatient clinic, the name "Somers" is printed as clearly as on his patient's file. And doesn't a single name come with a coherent body? (pp. 62–63)

Here Mol provides us with an account of a physician forced into calibration. The diagnostic interview and the pressure tests do not align. Either there are two different patients, two different diseases, or the doctor must find a way to resolve the inconsistent findings. This is an act of ontological calibration. The physician must find a way to link the findings of the diagnostic inventory with the findings of the pressure test.

In a strikingly similar presentation before the MPG, a pain management physician highlights the benefits physical therapists can offer in terms of diagnosis and patient assessment. The presenter works to link (calibrate) the situated functional evaluations of patient activity offered by physical therapists to the structural (anatomical) assessments of MDs:

And of course from a medical standpoint, we are good at looking at bodily structures and functions. We can look at pain, anxiety, range of motion, strength, endurance, all of these medical symptoms that the medical system is pretty good at evaluating and coming up with if there is a disease process that is involved in this. The functional capacity evaluation can actually be somewhat helpful in looking at our activities or how we perform these activities despite these bodily disorders and functions. Functional capacity evaluation, for those who don't know, are basically a list of tasks that a physical therapist is trained to look at and see if a patient is able to do this properly or with enough reserve so that they don't hurt themselves. So, there are certain tasks that physical therapists will be able to say, "Yeah, that person can sit for eight hours, stand for eight hours, or push two hundred pounds of whatever; can climb on ladders, can walk and use stairs." So these are pretty discrete tasks that a physical therapist can accurately say that a patient can or cannot do those activities. But again, we know that certain disease processes or certain pain issues can influence a person's ability to function or carry out their activities. But a lot of times, if we look at the big picture, basically if you look at patients with chronic back pain, we have all these things that physicians are really good at looking at. Here, we have activities that physical therapists are very good at looking at too. And we can say whether a person's performance is actually matching up to their capacity to do work. (MPG Journal Club, April 2006)

Whereas the technician in Mol's account aims to coordinate biomechanical measures with patient subjective report, the metadiscursive activity of the MPG offers the grounds upon which such calibrations can be made. By explicitly offering an account of the limits of biomechanical testing and creating a space whereby the functional evaluations of physical therapists can contribute productively to comprehensive care, the presenter authorizes future extradisciplinary practice. No longer does the internist need to fall back on disciplinary silos and paradigmatic justifications. When next he or she confronts a complex pain patient, multimodal treatment is authorized.

In *The Body Multiple*, Mol outlines two primary means of ontological calibration, activities she dubs simply "adding up" and "calibrating" (p. 84). Adding up happens more often, especially when the conflict is between subjective patient report and objective laboratory assessment. Diagnostic data is collected. The epistemological hierarchy of medical science is invoked, and untrusted data is discarded. In the case above, the pressure test is true, and the patient report is false. A second mode of adding up ignores conflict. Clinicians collect as many data points from as many different ontologies as possible. The subsequent decision is made through scorekeeping. Whichever possible result has the most data is the correct answer, and an appropriate treatment plan is developed. Adding up is a practical form of calibration. The doings of doctors manage the conflicting ontologies through hierarchy or scorekeeping. However, Mol also articulates a space for a model of calibration more in keeping with the practices of rhetorical inquiry.

Continuing with the case of conflicting test outcomes, Mol outlines calibration as follows:

> If test outcomes were listened to as if they were each speaking for themselves alone, they might get confined within different paradigms. The question whether different tests say the same thing or rather something different would not be answerable—indeed it could hardly be asked. The possibility to negotiate between clinical notes, pressure measurements numbers, duplex graphs, and angiographic images arises thanks to the correlation studies that actively make them comparable with one another. The threat of incommensurability is countered in practice by establishing common measures. Correlation studies allow for the possibility (never friction free) of translations. (pp. 84–85)

Here we see calibration is a sort of meta-activity. In fact, it's so meta that in Mol's study it only gets a quick mention as something that happens in correlation studies. The details of these studies are beyond the scope of Mol's analysis. As a rhetorician, it is precisely spaces like these studies that interest me. The work of calibration is predicated on the metapractical discourse of correlation. How do different diagnostic ontologies get calibrated? How are the different forms of diagnostic practice realigned, reinterpreted, rearticulated so that they may "speak" to each other, so that translation may occur? For Mol, this is a black box—a black box I aim to unpack. As I suggest above, the MPG functions in a rather similar fashion to Mol's correlation studies. It is a metapractical space where discussants can calibrate divergent ontologies. It is a space where they can ask questions about practical, epistemological, and metaphysical conflicts that will enable practical calibration in clinical settings.

Ontological calibration is the "what." The next pressing question is "how?" In this chapter, I have sketched out the basic shape of the MPG and its representational practice. I have outlined the presentational genres (article summary, article synthesis, basic science presentation, and practice reflection) and deliberative practices (off-label discussion) that stage ontological calibration. In so doing, I hope to have offered a compelling exigency for rhetorical-ontological inquiry as the study of the (representational) practices devoted to the adjudication of clinical practices and emergent ontologies. Ultimately, I believe practices like calibration, adding up, and other similar acts of representation yet to be identified constitute the essential contribution of spaces like the MPG and the methodological core of rhetorical-ontological inquiry. In the next chapter, I extend my inquiry into ontological calibration by exploring how the calibrating practices of the MPG serve to create and authorize the new nonmodern pain ontologies that the MPG members hope will proliferate. In so doing, I will bring rhetorical-ontological inquiry closer to traditional rhetorical territory by investigating how particular discursive structures circulate within the broader ecology of practices from calibrating to clinical. Ultimately, the anchor point for this discussion will be a modification of the rhetorical theory of stasis—the stopping points in discourse where prior questions must be deliberated as the foundation for future action.

CHAPTER THREE

Ontological Calibration and Functional Stases in the MPG

Followed while being enacted [disease] multiplies—for practices are many. But the ontology that comes with equating what is with what is done is not of a pluralist kind. The many-foldedness of objects enacted does not imply their fragmentation. Although atherosclerosis in the hospital comes in different versions, these somehow hang together. . . . The drawing together of a diversity of objects that go by a single name involves various modes of calibration. —Annemarie Mol, *The Body Multiple*

[The MPG] creates a fuller picture of what pain is. You appreciate the complexity of the suffering as it relates to the patient's whole world. The complex pharmacology, the social interactions . . . it's kind of hard to describe. It's not an easy thing. Everybody's got a knowledge base that they can give you. . . . It has helped because you interact with other specialists who are interested in pain—physiologists, pharmacologists, basic scientists from the universities, attorneys, psychologists. And what I see is a mosaic of pain. When you sit in a group like that and start to put all the pieces of the mosaic together, you start to see the whole picture. The impact on the psychology, the basic science, the attorneys that deal with patients caught in a vortex of [legal and disability issues]. —Midwest Pain Group president

The above epigraphs juxtapose Mol's description of ontological calibration with the last serving MPG president Dr. Bennetti's reflection on its discourse. As Mol suggests and Dr. Bennetti's description of the MPG enacts, in cases of cross-ontological alignment, members of apparently conflicted ontologies do not run into the communicative brick wall that incommensurability theory predicts. Rather, there can be a process of aligning two or more preexisting ontologies and establishing a new hybrid practical-discursive space. Certainly in the case of the MPG, members' commitment to a nonmodern approach to pain management led them to establish the cross-ontological dialogue described in the above epigraph and preceding chapter. As the participants in this conversation establish a dialogue, their discussions become a negotiation between different practices and emergent metaphysics, a negotiation that can serve to establish and legitimize a new ontology. As such, the driving question for this chapter has to do with the rhetorical mechanisms whereby the members of the MPG calibrate monodisciplinary ontologies to enact a hybrid nonmodern approach to pain. In exploring this issue, I will draw on theoretical resources from diverse sources, from contemporary STS to classical rhetorical theory. Ultimately, this chapter argues that the MPG's work of ontological calibration can be understood through a functional adaptation of rhetorical stasis theory.

Functional Stasis Theory

In the case of the MPG, the stasis questions are powerful moments of ontological calibration. These stases allow the MPG to articulate their disagreement with the preexisting pain ontologies established in the individual's monodisciplinary practice and additionally serve as strategies for calibration and the subsequent establishment of a new nonmodern ontology. As Heidlebaugh (2001) argued, such stasis points are the opportunity where a discussant can "use what she has before her to suggest the beginnings of new positions (or new systems, new narratives)" (p. 145). As members of the MPG explore stasis questions, they begin to forge a new, shared ontology of pain that exceeds or escapes the conflicting discourses of their monodisciplinary ontologies. Furthermore, as they explore a whole host of stasis questions, they describe the institutional obstacles to ontological change and the possibilities and limits of agency. This function of stasis doctrine enacts the balance that McKeon (1966) ascribes to communication as it "provide[s] both the initial definition of problems and the dynamism of their evolution" (p. 93).

As it is typically understood, Quintilian's taxonomy of stases represents inquiry primarily into rational and legal questions (Walker, 2000, p. 61). The rational stases in this system—which include *stochamos* (conjectural), questions dealing with issues of fact or existence, *horos* (definitional) that concern the name that should be applied to a fact, and *symbebekos* (circumstantial or qualitative)—are concerned with contingencies of judgment. To these stases, McKeon and Gross, following Cicero, add a fourth: *metalepsis* or "translative" stases concerned with the question of jurisdiction and appropriate venue or body of experts making a judgment (McKeon, 1966, p. 371; McKeon, 1987, p. 62; Gross, 2004, p. 142; Gross, 2005, p. 181). In recent work, however, stasis theory has been applied to all kinds of discourse (Kennedy, 1983, p. 85), and contemporary uses of stasis theory by McKeon, Prelli, and Gross make stasis relevant to any discourse where claims are in dispute. While Gross has applied stasis theory to the invention of new scientific theory, and Koerber (2006a) considered the role of stasis in the evolution of pediatric medicine and its evaluation of the immune function of breast milk, Prelli's (2005) use of stasis in scientific controversy was perhaps its most thorough application to scientific discourse. Prelli developed a system of superior and subordinate stases and argues that in science, stasis points can provide a foundation for multidisciplinary communication:

> *Stasis* questions can operate as "reference points" where controversialists can enter each other's perspective and, thereby, discern their similarities and differences. . . . *Stasis* questions furnish potential sites for transforming controversy into collaboration. They can function as loci for negotiating new grounds in common for addressing particular, situated problems of mutual concern. (p. 303)

Thus, stases are the standing point or stopping point at which argument commences and where ontological calibration often begins.

Prelli augments the classical stasis repertoire by adding a suite of superior stases—evidential, interpretive, evaluative, and methodological. To this taxonomy, Graham and Herndl (2011) add a "practical" superior stasis in order to account for interrupting questions addressing issues of technical praxis that fall outside the laboratory. For both Prelli and Graham and Herndl, superior stases coordinate with the classical or "inferior" stases to provide a sixteen-point (for Prelli) or twenty-point (for Graham and Herndl) taxonomy of stases—the methodological-qualitative, the practical-conjectural, and so on. Such taxonomies provide very useful ways to explore the nature of stases in the course of debate. Prelli describes the evidential-translative stasis as determining "which from among alternative bodies of data and evidence provides the best criteria for resolving evidential problems" (Prelli, 2005, p. 306). Furthermore, my prior work with Carl Herndl (2011) (which addresses a data set that overlaps with this chapter) offers a clear explanation of the work of this new compound stasis in the discourse of the MPG:

> Clinical experience tells the members of the MPG that much of their practice works, that they have impacts, but the evidence is not recognized. Research into and treatment of pain requires heavy reliance on subjective patient report.

However, this reliance on subjectivity is in direct conflict with the broader project of Western science and its pursuit of objectivity. (p. 157)

While the evidential-translative stasis provides a good starting point for
thinking about stasis moments in the MPG, I aim to push beyond a taxonomic stasis analysis. While I could provide a sixteen- or twenty-point
taxonomic analysis (à la Prelli, 2005, or Graham & Herndl, 2011) of the key
issues in the MPG discourse, I offer what I think will be a more fruitful approach: a *functional* stasis analysis. In making this distinction, I'm taking
a cue from neuroimaging scientists. Neurologists differentiate between
structural and functional imaging studies. Structural imaging seeks to describe the anatomy of the brain. It identifies prominent neuroanatomical
features and locates them relative to other features. It is concerned with
a cartography of the brain—where does one structure begin and another
end? In contrast, functional imaging studies work to describe physiology.
How do blood and oxygen flow through various brain features as they
process information and stimuli? Structural imaging is three-dimensional;
functional imaging is four-dimensional—gathering data over time. I
would argue that the typical taxonomic approach to stasis theory is structural—it isolates individual stases from the flow of argument. In contrast,
functional stasis analysis seeks to capture the dynamic and often nested
relationship among stases within the flow of debate. This allows the analysis to more effectively address the multi-ontological complexity of MPG
debate. Additionally, functional stasis analysis, in tracking the flow of stases in situ, allows for the interrogation of the resolution of stasis questions
into new topoi that will be deployed as calibration proceeds.

Stases at the MPG

In a move that inadvertently (I presume) replicates the dictates of stasis theory, the MPG has developed a conversation that offers members
the opportunity to explore the points of contradiction separating the
discourse of the traditional pain configurations from the discourse they
would like to create. During their off-label discussions, members of the
MPG engage in a self-reflexive conversation about their professional languages and the limitations these languages impose on practice and research. These metapractical moments occur following presentations, in
the discussion portion of the evening when members engage in a dialogue

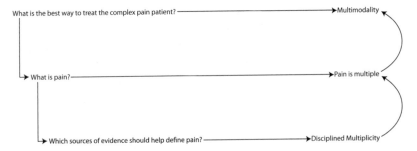

FIGURE 3.1. Functional stasis mapping of the MPG discourse, detailing the interactive nested stases, topical resolutions, and buttressing that occur in the calibrating discourse of the MPG.

that explores not only nontraditional treatments but also their collective frustration with reductive ontologies of pain staged by the isolated clinical practices.

My analysis of these activities at the MPG has identified four primary stases central to their work of ontological calibration. A structural stasis analysis following Prelli and Graham and Herndl would identify these stases as (1) practical-qualitative, (2) interpretive-definitive, (3) evidential-translative, and (4) practical-translative. And while these constructs will provide useful insights as my analysis progresses, my primary concern is with the functional aspects of situated stases. As such, I will begin my exploration with a functional mapping of three of these stases (see fig. 3.1). (The analysis of the fourth identified stasis falls outside the flow of this argument and will be revisited in the penultimate section of this chapter.)

In keeping with the functional mode of analysis, figure 3.1 focuses primarily on the relationship between stases, and between stases and topoi, rather than a taxonomy of static forms. Within this model, three static "physiological" functions are evident: nesting, resolution, and buttressing. I use *nesting* to describe the particular relationship among stases that occurs when positing one stasis question forces discussants to address a second, prior stasis. The latter stasis is said to be nested in the former, and I have represented this with the arrows on the left-hand side that drop and then turn at a ninety-degree angle to the right. In the sections that follow, I will explore in greater detail how each stasis nests into the next, but for the moment, I hope the suggestion that questions about proper treatment must rely on questions about disease definition will suffice. *Resolution* occurs when the argumentative processes of stasis debate come to a close—that is, when an answer is provided. (Resolutions are represented in fig. 3.1 with straight arrows.) Rhetorically, I understand these static resolutions to be the establishment of new topoi—new common places—for future discussion/praxis. Praxiographically, I understand resolutions to be calibration in action. When stasis questions are resolved, so too is the cross-ontological conflict. (Of course, resolution need not always be agreeable for everyone. It may take the form of subordination, as in Mol's adding up.) Lastly, I use the term *buttressing*—represented in figure 3.1 by the curvilinear arrows to the right—to refer to the interaction between nested topic resolutions and higher-order stases. That is, when stases nest, the resolution of the infrastases is required for the resolution of the suprastases. The newly established topos at the lower level buttresses the soon-to-be established topos at the higher level.

First-Order Stasis: Practical-Qualitative

My first order of stasis analysis harkens back to the origin of the MPG as well as the biopsychosocial metaphysics of pain. As one might expect from clinicians, the first stasis and exigency for nonmodernity is rooted primarily in clinical practice. However, many MPG members reported that the decision to join the MPG and engage in interdisciplinarity did not necessarily come easily. Indeed, the members of the MPG rejected the hegemony of any single discipline (including their own) and embraced a multidisciplinary perspective. This is a major shift for individuals who have been through four to eight years of formal health-care education and up to ten additional years of apprenticeships, residencies, fellowships, and board certifications. In fact, members of the MPG sometimes refer to these recognitions about the limitedness of their home disciplines and methods and the value of others as a "conversion experience" or an "epiphany."[1]

MPG members consistently reported during subject interviews that these epiphanies arose from dissatisfaction with monodisciplinary practice. Specifically, MPG clinicians encountered complex pain patients for whom a single pain ontology was an insufficient basis for treatment. For example, MPG founder Dr. Peters reflected about the early days of his practice and his sense that there should be more to offer patients:

> When we started we were very opiate focused. But we'd get hugely complex patients, patients with psychological problems and liver failure. We were writing a lot of opiate scripts early on, but it wasn't enough. Now we use multidisciplinary

interventions, psych, chiropractic, other interventions. [Opiate prescription] is a tool, but it's not the answer. (Peters, ethnographic interview)

In this passage, Peters retraces the evolution of his practice from mono-disciplinary within the biochemical ontology to something more hybrid. However, he glosses over the actual conversion portion of the experience. How does that happen?

An interview with gerontologist Dr. Olsen sheds some light on the issue. In speaking about his experience with his own health history, he identifies how a local site of practice centered around a complex patient (in this case Dr. Olsen himself) can foster a nonmodern epiphany:

> I think some of the people we have [at the MPG] are on the edge [when it comes to adopting the hybrid approach]. . . . Through that, through seeing improvements, where an orthopedic surgeon has had failure, but they see improvement [their patients had with a clinician from another discipline] and they think to themselves, "Well, shit, maybe there is something there." I suffer from degenerative-disc disease and spinosus. It forced me to exercise a lot and do something that's beyond pills and surgery. I've met a lot of swimmers who are physicians, and I ask them, "What are you doing here?" And they say, "I've exhausted all the other avenues for pain control, so now I swim, and I go see a chiropractor for my back." They've had a conversion experience based on their own personal health history. And I think that is one way to get into the different integrative areas complementing one another, but working together and seeing patient improvement is another way. There's a lot of stuff you wonder about the merit of it, but there's a trend, you see an improvement in the quality of life. (Olsen, ethnographic interview)

The recognition that pain patients are suffering in ways that transcend monodisciplinary practice opens up the first stasis issue of my analysis: if patients are complex, then what are the best ways to treat them? Dr. Olsen recounts how this question encouraged him to search for answers beyond the scope of his own practice and training. Allopathic medicine is generally pretty hostile to chiropractic medicine. However, the local site of practice provided a reason to question (stasis) the monodisciplinary scope of practice.

Indeed, addressing such practical-qualitative issues was often cited as a primary rationale for and source of satisfaction with the MPG. Physician's assistant Hamlyn highlighted how potential success with improving patient health contributes to a greater awareness and acceptance of extra-disciplinary treatment options for members of the MPG:

> I think that the enthusiasm that the members of the MPG have for the treatment of patients with pain is very inspiring for those of us that do this day to day. Because it is a difficult and challenging role to try to help these patients that have a variety of factors that are contributing to their pain beyond just the physical malady. I think with enough people and diverse fields approaching patients with pain, we're much more apt to be successful. If we look at it in terms of a team approach with the goal of lessening an individual's pain, and seeing it as a team rather than opposition among the different modalities and disciplines as they treat an individual in pain, it will in the future be more successful overall. (Hamlyn, ethnographic interview)

Though Hamlyn is prognostic whereas Olsen is reflective, they both articulate the goal of improved health with multidisciplinary clinical practice. Indeed, Olsen and Hamlyn were not the only interviewees who, when asked why they joined the MPG, responded with a variant of "because I was interested [in] improving the management of pain" (Boysen, ethnographic interview).

The recognition of a practical-qualitative stasis is not only motivational. It also constitutes a locus of ontological calibration. In exploring various modes of practice, the members of the MPG work to create a space for ontological multiplicity and a recognition of its value. For example, in a presentation on chiropractic techniques for managing back pain, the original speaker shared research regarding a series of techniques that patients can do on their own at home, without the aid of a clinician. In response, Dr. Heisenberg, a neurologist, pointed to a lack of easy-to-read pamphlets that could guide patients through such techniques. This question sparked a dialogue that worked to calibrate chiropractic medicine, physical therapy, and psychology:

DR. HEISENBERG (NEUROLOGIST): This is one of the challenges I've always found. It is that these articles are published, but very infrequently do they publish a booklet or pamphlet that I can then immediately apply. There probably is in chiropractor groups places where these exercises are readily available. But I find that a little lacking in our profession.

DR. NELSON (PHYSICAL THERAPIST): Physical therapists actually have a very good idea on how to implement these. I would refer [patients] to physical therapists since I know you guys have a lot more contacts with physical therapists. But since I just started my practice, please send everyone to me.

DR. GREEN (PSYCHOLOGIST): I want to raise a question with this. I'm going to talk about a study from Stanford that has to do with treating high blood pressure with relaxation exercises. He did this really impressive study where the two groups of patients have relaxation training. One group, you handed the people the tape and the tape recorder and you sent them home to practice. The other [group], the therapist sat down and went through the exercise with them, and then gave the tape recorder and sent them to practice. . . . But it was just the group that had the therapist instruction that had the dramatic drop in blood pressure. . . . And the group that you just give the tape to and send home and they do the exercises, didn't get any better. I think in this kind of thing, when you think about just giving someone a pamphlet and sending them home, we can't assume that that's equivalent treatment to sending them to a therapist, be it a physical therapist or whatever, to instruct them in the exercises individually. I think there is some psychological impact to that part of the treatment that we often don't realize. I've had physicians call me as say, "Would you give this guy a relaxation tape?" Well, no, I don't do that, because I've got a little bit of data here that suggests that's not very efficacious treatment. (MPG Journal Club, February 2007)

In the first response, we can see Dr. Nelson working to align the pain and the treatment options (practices) of chiropractors with those of physical therapists. Certainly, he is working in an economic mode and seeking to build his practice, but he is also linking an additional practical regime to the one explored in the formal presentation.

Although Dr. Green's comment may seem to be, in part, an act of boundary enforcement (and therefore an invocation of the translative stasis)—he will not give out tapes or pamphlets because patients need his special expertise (or more cynically, because he wants their money)—he also is completing an act of qualitative calibration in that it coordinates a study of psychological practice to the regimes of practice of chiropractors and physical therapists. In essence, he is saying that these clinicians have expertise and efficacious practices that cannot be reduced to tapes or pamphlets. In so doing, he supports the validity and utility of modes of practice other than his own. Of course, praxiographic subjects do not articulate their work and thought process using the lexicon of rhetorical-ontological inquiry. But in these passages we can see the practical-qualitative stasis shading immediately into the multimodal-practice topos. This is why a functional approach to stasis analysis is critical. It can better account not only for how the first-order stasis resolves, but also for the underlying logics and broader discourses that are tacitly folded into that resolution. In these short interview excerpts, it's easy to see a quick static resolution. But the dense rhetorical activity of the MPG demonstrates that that resolution is predicated on a prior nested stasis—one of definition.

Second-Order Stasis: Interpretive-Definitive

As they reflect on the underlying practices that have led to the reductive definitions in their individual disciplines, members of the MPG develop a new interpretive-definitional stasis for pain. This stasis that emerges from their dialogue places the traditional two-world model of pain against the new hybrid approach for which the MPG is searching. This reflection also provides the MPG with opportunities to discuss the difficulty involved in formulating a new theory of pain that arises when the practical-translative stasis manifests in clinical settings. The initial locus of ontological calibration in the MPG actually originated outside of it, in the work of the IASP.

The official IASP (1994) definition of pain explicitly attempts to "represent agreement between diverse specialties including anesthesiology, dentistry, neurology, neurosurgery, neurophysiology, psychiatry, and psychology." The IASP's efforts to establish a broad definition and foster an integrated discourse on pain are both laudable and necessary. But establishing a working definition and a common discourse that enfranchises members of such widely differentiated disciplines and research traditions as neurosurgery and psychology is easier said than done. The IASP's Taskforce of Taxonomy is charged with creating a multidisciplinary definition of pain and pain-related medical language. Underscoring the varied approaches and understandings of pain, the IASP provides definitions of more than twenty pain-related terms, including pain types (e.g., neurogenic pain, allodynia, and peripheral neuropathic pain), pain "syndromes" (e.g., dysesthesia, hyperalgesia, and neuralgia), and pain-related terminology (nociceptor, noxious stimulus, and pain tolerance level). The entry for "pain," however, is one of its lengthiest and includes multiple explanatory notes that serve to emphasize the problematic nature of defining and assessing pain:

> An unpleasant sensory and emotional experience associated with actual or potential tissue damage, or described in terms of such damage. Note: The inability to communicate verbally does not negate the possibility that an individual

is experiencing pain and is in need of appropriate pain-relieving treatment. Pain is always subjective. Each individual learns the application of the word through experiences related to injury in early life. Biologists recognize that those stimuli which cause pain are liable to damage tissue. Accordingly, pain is that experience we associate with actual or potential tissue damage. It is unquestionably a sensation in a part or parts of the body, but it is also always unpleasant and therefore also an emotional experience. Experiences which resemble pain but are not unpleasant, e.g., pricking, should not be called pain. Unpleasant abnormal experiences (dysesthesias) may also be pain but are not necessarily so because, subjectively, they may not have the usual sensory qualities of pain.

Many people report pain in the absence of tissue damage or any likely pathophysiological cause; usually this happens for psychological reasons. There is usually no way to distinguish their experience from that due to tissue damage if we take the subjective report. If they regard their experience as pain and if they report it in the same ways as pain caused by tissue damage, it should be accepted as pain. This definition avoids tying pain to the stimulus. Activity induced in the nociceptor and nociceptive pathways by a noxious stimulus is not pain, which is always a psychological state, even though we may well appreciate that pain most often has a proximate physical cause. (IASP, 1994)

Despite its thoroughly multidisciplinary nature, the IASP's definition underscores the difficulty that can arise in multi-ontological calibration as the second paragraph almost directly contradicts the first.

Although pain is defined as subjective and emotional, and the definition takes great care to divorce the medical understanding of pain from a physical mechanism of injury, the link to physical stimuli is ever present. The definition directly relates the subjective-emotional experience to "actual or potential tissue damage," "descrip[tion] in terms of such damage," and "injury in early life." Pain is explicitly described as physical in the statement, "It is *unquestionably* a sensation in part or parts of the body." Yet at the same time, the definition works against this physically grounded conception of pain, stating that pain is "emotional," "always subjective," "learn[ed]," "not identical with "nociception," and "*always* psychological." The multiplicity of pain does not resolve in the IASP definition, which is a primary origin point for the nonmodern ontology. This is uncomfortable, but perhaps necessary.

The MPG's more local efforts to calibrate biochemical and psychological pain ontologies often follow the same logic of multiplicity as the IASP definition. The interpretive-definitional discourse aims to grapple with that multiplicity without being reductive. For example, in the following excerpt from a discussion over the nature of "empathetic pain," Dr. Kapplan attempts to determine whether or not the authors of a particular paper, presented by his colleague Dr. Landau, were operating within a dualist metaphysics:

> This is very interesting, more from a philosophical point of view than a science point of view. I was trying to, as you were presenting this, trying to see if they were dualist or nondualist from a philosophical point of view. Was your impression that the authors were more dualist, that there's two separate things—a mind and a body—or that they weren't dualist in terms of that? And also, the problem I have with dualism is that there has to be that magical thinking point . . . there is something happening there that can't be identified, and that you can't put a finger on. So I have an inherent problem with a dualist philosophy impinging upon neurophysiology because of that difficulty there, that you always have that step you can never identify. (MPG Journal Club, November 2006)

The "magical thinking point" that Dr. Kapplan identifies as his problem with dualism is an avatar of traditional critiques of empiricism based on mental perceptions of physical stimuli. More to the point, it echoes, unintentionally no doubt, Latour's metaphor of the "mind-in-a-vat"—the philosopher's caustic dismissal of modern empiricism and its epistemological dilemmas as a dualism, a mind isolated in a vat, that nevertheless is required to generate certain knowledge of the physical world outside it (Latour, 1999, p. 4). For both Latour and Dr. Kapplan, this leaves something, a cognitive or metaphysical something, you can't put your finger on.

This "something you can't put your finger on" is of great concern to some in the medical community. Indeed, even among those who advocate for something like a new nonmodern approach to pain, the IASP definition can be unsatisfactory, precisely because of the way it attempts to handle the dualisms rendered by the two-world problem. During an interview session with Dr. Michelson, an orthopedist from the AAPM, I asked what he thought of the IASP definition, expecting support. Instead, he responded:

> I ignore it as much as I can, because it obscures the difference between perception and experience. There's no way to reconcile these two uses of the word, unless you acknowledge they are separate and that one is objective and one

is subjective. You're lost using the same word to describe two entirely different events—neurobiologically and phenomenologically. Until the study of pain
clearly separates the objective from the subjective. I disagree [with the IASP].
Here's the paradox of my position: it makes me sound like a dualist. That I'm
creating a dual nature of pain, when I think the people that try to integrate
them, they are the neo-dualists who think that thinking and feeling are fundamentally separate.

While I certainly agree that Dr. Michelson's objections to the IASP definition make him sound like a dualist, the definition he eventually arrives
at is remarkably similar to multiple ontologies, and thus warrants con-
sideration here. When confronted with the interpretive-definitive stasis,
Dr. Michelson rejects its premise. He argues that pain is very clearly defined under the transmission-communication model and suggests that
pain management clinicians need to address not pain but the phenomenology of suffering. Under this rubric, Michelson defines suffering as a
"threat or perceived threat to the autobiographical self" (Michelson, ethnographic interview). This, of course, sounds like a form of postmodern
medicine that reifies the disease/illness dichotomy, and to a certain extent
it is. However, since Dr. Michelson defines the autobiographical self in
terms of lived experience—that is, something that is born of embodied
doings in the world, I would argue that despite his dualist construction
of subjective versus objective, he nevertheless ends up with an approach
to pain and suffering that is similar to early efforts at establishing a nonmodern approach to inquiry (see, for example, Latour, 1993; or Haraway,
1991, 1997).

In any event, unresolved conflicts over defining pain is a recurrent
topic of MPG conversation and becomes a point of stasis for its members'
developing discourse as they try to establish a language adequate to their
practice of pain management. MPG members often alternate between
referring to pain as a "phenomenon" and a "problem," and they modify
these terms with adjectives like "complex" and "multidimensional." Furthermore, MPG members use metaphors like "puzzle" (Fitzpatrick, ethnographic interview) and "mosaic" (Bennetti, ethnographic interview) to
refer to the problems associated with and processes involved in assem-
bling all the various conceptions of pain into a single definition. Perhaps
the clearest example of the MPG angst surrounding the problem of pain
comes from a follow-up to the interview with Landau referenced in my
introduction. After calling for a new Freud, Landau argues:

There is a major cognitive shift going to happen with the mind-body connection, and somebody who's a real good synthesizer is going to put it together in a way that is strongly supported by science. And we're going to be able to make a big jump in pain treatment, because there's no model out there right now. They can put it together, and put it together without all the bias and prejudice that frankly started with Descartes. (Landau, ethnographic interview)

Dr. Peters, the founder of the MPG, describes the common experience of pain and the troubling difficulty defining it:

There are various definitions of pain: unpleasant sensation that can be an actual or potential damage as the IASP says "as described in terms of such damage." We all know what pain is. It is like when I think it was Oliver Wendell Holmes who said, "I know what pornography is, I just can't describe it." It is like that with pain. You know it when you see it. I think all of us know what pain is. We all can understand what it means when people say they are in horrible pain. We can think back on our lives to a time when we were in pain. But it is a very difficult thing to define. It's like other things in our life. Like love. These things are not easy to define although we may know [them]. (Peters, ethnographic interview)

Here pain is both actual damage to bodily tissue, "as described in terms of such damage," and an unpleasant sensation. The definition is elusive, like pornography or love. Peters struggles to recognize both the physical element of pain, the damage, and the emotional or subjective experience of it. Replicating the logic of praxiography, he suggests that our "understanding" of pain is, finally, grounded in personal experience and memory; when we hear someone talk about their pain, our understanding emerges from recollections of our own experience.

As MPG members struggle to rationalize their divergent clinical practices and calibrate diverse ontologies, they confront the contradictions within the new, multidisciplinary discourse on pain that the IASP is explicitly attempting to facilitate. This self-reflective conversation not only allows members of the MPG to reflect on the philosophical problems that plague contemporary science and medicine; it leads them toward definitions of pain that calibrate the biochemical and psychological ontologies. Periodically, MPG members attempt boundary-crossing definitions of pain that address the interpretive-definitional stasis. For example, Dr. Landau, in the discussion on pain empathy from which I have already quoted, said:

> The activity in the pain network is sensitive to the top-down perceptual process. The mental representation of nociception in the pain experience results from the interaction between noxious sensory input and cognitive factors. (MPG Journal Club, November 2006)

While Landau's language is more technical than Peters's, the same difficulty emerges from her analysis. Landau needs to find a way of combining the nociceptive and psychological components of pain. In so doing, she articulates their relationship hierarchically (top-down), on the one hand, and temporally ("pain experience" that "results"), on the other. Indeed, this might be a moment where calibration and adding up intersect. Landau places different ontologies of pain in a hierarchy that could be used for cross-ontological adjudication in practice. Dr. Fitzpatrick's presentation on fibromyalgia also uses the temporal link between stimulus and resulting experience to frame the interaction between the sensory and cognitive elements of pain:

> Nociceptive information is saying, "Boy, that's a strong stimulus. I've localized it to my shoulder." [It's] these characteristics. I know it is of such intensity, that it should hurt. But the cingulate gyrus and these other [brain] areas have to come in and add to it . . . to say, "And it hurts!" So when we think about pain, we always have to think about these two components: the nociceptive, which is simply the physiological processing of a bit of sensory information, and then the context or association we put to it. Does it hurt? I.e., that's what makes it pain—the two things together. (MPG Journal Club, February 2008)

Here pain is explicitly a hybrid comprised of "a bit of sensory information" and an emotional context ("Does it hurt?").

As a final example of how members of the MPG work at definitional calibration, I offer a presentation of the epidemiology and etiology of migraine headaches by pain physician Dr. Heisenberg. He begins an argument for the integration of a vast multitude of factors into the understanding of migraines by showing a schematic representation of migraines as a theoretical concept. The polar-plot-like diagram he provides depicts migraines as an integrated phenomenon at the intersection of the physical axes of head pain. But his depiction also includes nausea, cold hands, fatigue, despondency, and flatulence among others elements of migraine pain. Heisenberg uses this slide to argue that medical practice needs to use the proper diagnostic inventories to assess not only the migraine but also the efficacy of treatment. He expresses serious concern that most of the questionnaires used in the literature (and in clinical practice) fail to address the cognitive-emotional aspects that are integral to migraines:

> So one of the things that is also an item of debate is which questionnaire to use. Oh gosh, does this sound familiar to psychologists? Which questionnaire should you use? There's actually an extraordinarily simple questionnaire called the HIT-6, and we haven't brought that to the group for a while, but that was promulgated by Glaxo. But nonetheless, it covers all areas of function. MIDAS actually only covers a few . . . it doesn't really cover energy. It doesn't ask you cognition questions. You, as a clinician, actually have to imply that in your questioning. It's kind of good to talk to the patient, besides just having them fill out a form. And emotional distress isn't covered. The most commonly used study methodology when determining severity of migraine disability is actually [MIDAS], in almost all the studies that are published now, even though there are actually better questionnaires in terms of covering everything. So, we need to see some further developments along this line. (MPG Journal Club, February 2007)

Heisenberg objects to the dominant questionnaire, MIDAS, because it does not recognize the emotional and functional aspects of pain. The very next slide in his presentation, however, reduces migraines to a function of the descending nucleus of five—a biomechanical structure. In order to support his argument for the interactional nature of the physiological and psychological aspects of migraine pain, Heisenberg ultimately references physiology. As he outlines it, the brain structures that create the physiological dimension of migraine pain are close enough to those that create the psychological dimension that those "extra" psychological symptoms are present:

> If you look at the descending nucleus of five, the nucleus of pain is spread out over a space. It's not just a small group of cells. And unfortunately it is interweaved with this lower portion of the nucleus, which are actually inputs from the back of the head for sensation and pain. Also very close by are nuclei that control [sinus- and congestion-related] symptoms. So it's easy to understand why we get so many of these look-alike syndromes in migraines. The point of all this is most of what we call the "extra features" of migraines are not actually covered well in these studies. What is covered only [are] the diagnostic categories. (MPG Journal Club, February 2007)

What operates as a set of contradictions in the static discourse of the IASP appears as a series of stases for the MPG as their ongoing intellectual collaboration identifies points of conflict and disagreement. Dr. Fitzpatrick's claim that pain is "the two things together" is representative of the MPG's struggle to collapse the Cartesian dualism. Stasis analysis allows us to see the ongoing calibrating activity involved in the MPG's attempts to coordinate modernist clinical practices into nonmodern ontologies staged by multimodal pain science and practice.

Third-Order Stasis: Evidential-Translative

As my analysis suggests, members of the MPG struggle to calibrate the many pain ontologies that span the two-world problem and its correlative dualisms. Inventing a new definition adequate to their range of clinical practices is extremely difficult. As accidental autopraxiographers, the members of the MPG are comfortable with the hybrid ontology staged by their clinical practice. But despite their intentions, dualisms persist in the empirical-discursive ontology staged by evidence-based medicine in general and pain science in particular. All this presents a significant problem for many in health care. The authority of EBM and the ubiquity of randomized controlled trials as the dominant methodology confronts MPG members with a difficult problem: what data and what data-gathering methods are appropriate to their emerging pain ontologies? The short answer for the MPG, of course, is theirs—the MPG's own data collection. In fact, Dr. Bennetti even describes the developing mission of the MPG as an effort to become "a body of expert knowledge not within each little community but also within the state legislatively" (MPG Journal Club, May 2008). And, indeed, this would be an important concern if Dr. Peters, the MPG's founder, is correct in his assessment:

> There's a huge battle on the horizon between the pain physicians—interventionists [who prescribe opiates for pain] versus multimodal multidisciplinary approach [such as that explored by the MPG]. Has to do with payment and salary. (Peters, ethnographic interview)

Dr. Peters's concerns about remuneration highlight the material expression of the evidential-translative stasis explored by the members of the MPG. The reconstitution of pain within a nonmodern ontology staged by both diverse clinical practices and data from RCTs opens the jurisdictional stasis typically closed off by the firm disciplinary and legal structures of Western biomedicine. Who decides what data are legitimate? Who enforces discursive regulations that shape resolving topoi?

MPG members recognize that some knowledge emerges from clinical practice in qualitative forms that are not typically recognized by the rationality that dominates regulatory agencies and insurance-industry analyses. As the MPG explores the interpretive-definitional stasis, they confront the evidential-translative stasis that is nested in the former. When it comes to the questions of whose definition of pain is most relevant or whose approach to data is more valid, the particular stasis at issue is the jurisdictional (the translative). As Prelli (2005) describes it:

> *Translative* issues locate points for decision in questions about the relative appropriateness of alternative possible criteria, standards or "grounds" for acting upon problems of 1) existence (evidential), 2) meaning (interpretive), 3) significance (evaluative), 4) action (methodological). (pp. 307–308, emphasis in original)

In the data presented thus far, one can see how, when it comes to the definition of pain, these translative questions intersect with the definition—for example, which discipline's conception of pain is most valid: those with a biochemical ontology, those with a psychological ontology, or those with a nonmodern ontology?

Jurisdictional issues surround all four of Prelli's "superior stases" (evidential, interpretive, evaluative, and methodological) with regard to questions concerning the proper foundation for the science of pain. As previously noted, research into and treatment of pain requires heavy reliance on subjective patient report. However, this reliance on subjectivity is in direct conflict with the broader project of Western science and its foundations in supposed objectivity. Indeed, this is a point of great lament for MPG members. As she struggles with the "magical thinking point" Dr. Kapplan identifies in dualist definitions of pain, Dr. Landau comments:

> We have things we know—the things that people do that have an impact. There's lots of studies on belief and how that impacts on a physical illness. And we have no way of measuring that, in my opinion. We can't measure it. We know it exists. We can't measure it. (MPG Journal Club, November 2006)

Where Dr. Peters observed that we know what pain is but can't define it, Dr. Landau rearticulates the point as a problem in disciplinary methodology; there are things we know, but we can't measure them. Such clinical experience is recognized by MPG members but not by the institutional professionals who administer EBM. EBM regulates what type of data and what methodologies are legitimate. And EBM is the mechanism that distributes jurisdiction to nonpractitioners in the insurance industry and regulatory agencies.

The problem of empirical measurement in the study of pain was highlighted as a major problem by a variety of MPG presentations and interviews. The interpretive-definitional stasis of the MPG frequently identified the lack of empirical techniques as a major barrier to the development of a new definition. In an interview, Dr. Boysen laments:

> I don't have a way of hooking someone up to a pain-o-meter. We can measure pain behavior, but pain behavior is obviously very personalized. I have to listen to what people are telling me. You can define nociception much easier. . . . [T]he science of pain management and the science of pain is tough. We really don't have a way of truly measuring pain. . . . We can measure the response of nociceptors, but that's not pain. (Boysen, ethnographic interview)

In response to this problem, clinicians and researchers have invested quite a bit of time, money, and research into the development of effective pain measures, but ultimately these are all questionnaires and inventories that must rely almost entirely on patient report. Indeed, the question of pain and quality-of-life inventories constitutes a further nested jurisdictional discourse of its own, with frequent debate over which inventory is most appropriate in which cases.

For example, Dr. Boysen also expressed concerns that the design of the patient pain inventories, while often useful for research design, are not necessarily appropriate for clinical practice:

> I think the chronic pain literature is improving, but much of the older literature uses either the visual-analog scale or the 1–10 scale for pain, and I know why they do it; because you can easily do statistics and get a statistically significant change with an intervention. What is not done very often is a clinically significant change. I think that the chronic pain literature, what I would like to see it go towards is more functional scales or quality-of-life scales. (Boysen, ethnographic interview)

In this excerpt, we see a prime example of how evidential-translative issues can serve as points of stoppage within pain management discourse.

The practices of medical science and EBM stage an ontology where only objectively quantifiable sources of data are appropriate to research and practice. However, the MPG as a would-be expert body wants recognition for alternative sources of data, including subjective report and clinical experience. This creates a host of difficult-to-resolve jurisdictional issues that can be explored under Prelli's rubric. Evidentially, it raises the issue of what types of data can be considered—or treated as existent. Questions concerning pain and quality-of-life inventories point to a conflict over the appropriate interpretive schemata for this already-questioned data. And, of course, "significance" takes on a double meaning within evidence-based medicine and the subsequent hegemony of the randomized clinical trial. Within the collected recordings of MPG Journal Club meetings, I have hours of discussion pertaining to the importance and appropriateness of research findings as measured by statistical significance and power.

Returning to figure 3.1, we can see how my three orders of nested stases co-articulate and resolve into topoi that buttress further resolutions. The practical quandary of how to treat complex patients forces a reimagining of the definition of pain, which further requires confronting the question of what sources of data are appropriate to this new definition. The intersecting ontologies of multimodal pain management and EBM force a provisional resolution in the topos of disciplined multiplicity. MPG members' practices rely on subjective patient report. But to be calibrated appropriately, that report must be disciplined by the structures and practices of EBM—hence the proliferation of pain and quality-of-life inventories. Although the multiplicity of clinical and patient experiences are controlled and limited by these practices of statistical disciplining, that multiplicity is not elided or erased. Thus, the decision to provide a practical regime of engagement that allows for the incorporation of this data multiplicity serves to buttress the hybrid and conflicted definition of pain articulated by the IASP and elaborated by the MPG. Together the topoi of disciplined multiplicity and pain multiplicity further buttress the topos of multimodality—that is, multidisciplinary pain treatment practices. All told, these nested stases and topic resolutions constitute the discourse of ontological calibration that serves to establish the justification for the nonmodern ontology and provides the metapractical space for further calibration activities in situated practice. Unfortunately for the members of the MPG, however, the static work is never done. The internal calibrating activities that stage a nonmodern pain ontology force confrontation with the broader disciplinary and regulatory structures. The local calibration work of the MPG does not force global recognition of a new ontology. This brings me to the fourth stasis I have identified—one that nests from the entire static discourse of the functional mapping, but also transcends that mapping.

Unordered Stasis: Practical-Translative

This work with the MPG suggests that through the mechanism of EBM, regulatory institutions such as the DEA, the FDA, pharmaceutical companies, and the medical insurance industry exact as much, if not more, restrictive pressures on the ontology-stating clinical practices of the MPG than the different disciplines and their reductive definitions of pain. Data collected from the MPG underscores the fact that clinicians involved are keenly aware of the influences of regulatory agencies and insurance analysts and how they disrupt practice and research necessary to a new multidisciplinary pain science. MPG founder Dr. Peters, for example, is famous for his caricatures of HMO actuaries as satanic agents of evil. As has been well documented, the insurance industry has had a broader impact on the practice of medicine than the denial of care in individual cases (Scott, Ruef, Mendel & Caronna, 2000).

This demonization of insurance actuaries is based in large part on the pervasive sense, among MPG members, that those actuaries intrude in their practice. In withholding funding for certain procedures, they do not allow the clinicians to perform the treatment they feel is most warranted. Indeed, during many MPG meetings, I witnessed informal discussions on how to manage insurance actuaries. A common practice among MPG members was to identify the most medically necessary procedure as well as a far more expensive alternative. So, for example, an oncologist explained that if he needed a CT scan of the brain, he'd ask the insurance company for a full-body PET scan. When they said no, he'd say, "Well, I guess I can just do a CT scan of the brain." Apparently, the insurance actuaries would often agree to the cheaper procedure.

Although it was pervasive, the vilification of the insurance industry was not ubiquitous among MPG members. Academic physiologist Dr. Fitzpatrick offered a more conciliatory opinion in a follow-up interview:

A few years ago everybody and his brother were bemoaning the issues with HMOs and managed care. And the argument was, "These accountants were telling us how to practice medicine." Well, the accountants read the literature. All they were doing was saying, "Look, there's no support for doing this so we're not going to pay for it." So really, the modern era of evidence-based medicine was ushered in by the accountants in the managed-care scenario, third-party payers. To me it only makes sense. If there's no evidence that it works, then is it really wise to be spending a lot of money doing it? Or if there's evidence to show it doesn't work or maybe that it's harmful, then maybe we shouldn't be doing it. (Fitzpatrick, ethnographic interview)

Here Dr. Fitzpatrick entangles the unordered stasis with my third-order stasis. For him, the answer to the evidential-translative question is unambiguously EBM. Subsequently, he has a different frame of reference under which to evaluate the appropriateness of the actuarial role in clinical practice. It should be noted that Dr. Fitzpatrick is not a clinician. He does laboratory and pedagogical work in anatomy and physiology at an osteopathic medical school near the MPG. His practice stages the empirical-discursive discursive ontology. Thus, his emergent ontology does not make as much room for the epistemology of clinical experience. Nevertheless, this passage highlights the role of ongoing practical-translative stases in the MPG. It further exemplifies the complexity of nested stases. Although the practical-translative stasis is often presented as outside the nested stases of figure 3.1, the nuances of MPG discourse allow for the entanglement of one stasis question with another. Furthermore, I point to the ways in which clinical practice is accommodated to the economic structures of the health-insurance industry as prima facie evidence for the profound impact so-called discursive spaces can have on clinical practice. Despite Mol's compelling analysis, the practices that stage disease ontologies do not exist in a vacuum. They are controlled, influenced, and regulated by broader calibrating practices that exceed the local site of clinical doings.

Indeed, third-party payers are not the only institutions to influence ontology-staging clinical practices, particularly within the realm of pain medicine. DEA regulations provide another level of control for the use of opioid pharmacology. All clinicians who can write opioid prescriptions are issued an identification number from the DEA. Each prescription is tracked to ensure that it's not being filled at more than one pharmacy. Obviously this regulatory apparatus has been designed as a part of the war on drugs. Opioid diversion, or securing a legal prescription for opioids such as OxyContin and selling them to a third party, is pandemic in pain medicine. Indeed, Dr. Bennetti once remarked that "for every patient you catch diverting, there are two you missed" (MPG meeting, July 2007). As a result of widespread opioid abuse, the DEA has shifted some policing responsibilities to practicing clinicians. They can be held civilly and criminally liable if they have not taken adequate precautions to prevent opioid abuse and diversion. Indeed, this is such a central issue for MPG members that they enlisted an undercover agent on a joint local police department–DEA opioid diversion task force as a guest speaker. Citing that presentation, hospital pharmacist Dr. Benedict expands on his own role in investigating diversion:

> One of the more interesting presentations was with [the undercover agent] and the narcotic presentation, on diversion. Unfortunately, we have to work on cases in the hospital. Some of those spill out into the public. At a previous hospital [where I worked], prescription pads were stolen, and they were forged and used out in other retail pharmacies, which involved me helping find out what was going on. Knowing that there's a person that now I have contact with and maybe help get a problem solved a little sooner. (Benedict, ethnographic interview)

The policing requirements of clinical practice may be even more onerous. Active patient monitoring is a essential issue. Correspondingly, a June 2007 presentation to the MPG included visitors from a urinalysis lab that specializes in diversion. Physicians who contract with this lab regularly collect urine specimens from their patients and send them in. The lab has procedures to determine not only how much narcotic residue is in each urine sample, but how much should be based on prescription amount, drug type, patient weight and gender, and so on. Clinicians can then access longitudinal urinalysis data to help determine which and how many patients are diverting. In some cases, this was viewed as helpful. The clinicians saw it as a useful tool to help attend to the broader health (physiological and psychological) of the patient. In other cases, it was viewed as an expensive and onerous intrusion in clinical practice resulting from excessive DEA oversight. (And, of course, it's worth questioning the metaphysics of patient-hood staged by these regulatory-clinical practices. Recurrent urinalysis stages a patient metaphysics of criminality with potentially profoundly negative effects for patient outcomes.)

Much like in the case of securing the ideal treatment from insurance companies, clinicians also circumnavigated jurisdictional issues. For example, in the same meeting, MPG members noted that there are legal requirements for intervention and reporting if opioid patients test positively for marijuana. Subsequently, most MPG clinicians who contracted with a urinalysis service said they opt out of marijuana testing. If they don't know about it, the illegal drugs regulatory apparatus cannot go after them for not acting. Opioid qua valuable tool was a recurrent trope in the discourse of the MPG, as was the DEA's excessive influence. Indeed, there is a general sense in pain medicine more broadly that the war on drugs has damaged the ability to provide sound clinical care. Scholarly and popular press articles abound discussing the new climate of "opiophobia." Indeed, many primary-care physicians and local pharmacies have simply stopped prescribing or carrying opioids. This fact is used routinely as evidence that the DEA has become unreasonably intrusive. However, the climate of opiophobia is so pervasive that addressing the practical-translative stasis cannot happen within the clinic. MPG members recognize that it is a debate that must happen on the national regulatory stage.

During a 2006 meeting of the MPG, Dr. Peters sought to galvanize members to participate in the regulatory discussion surrounding what are known as "do not fill until" requirements. Many chronic pain patients undergo long-term opioid-based pain management. These patients have issues like intractable back pain. They are not going to get better; all they can do is manage the pain. Their conditions, despite being chronic, are often stable. However, in an effort to fight drug diversion, the DEA issued a ruling declaring that a patient must see a clinician for each and every schedule 2 prescription and that no opioid prescriptions can exceed a 30-day supply. This ruling caused great concern for MPG members on behalf of their chronic pain patients. According to MPG members, chronic pain patients who were not diversion risks did not need to see (and pay for) a clinical visit on a monthly basis. Pain clinicians nationwide petitioned the DEA for a reevaluation of the rule and were successful ("Issuance of Multiple Prescriptions," 2007). At the time of the aforementioned meeting, the DEA had issued a proposed revision whereby physicians could prescribe up to 90 days of narcotics in three separate prescriptions. The second and third would be limited under the "do not fill until" provision. The clinician could specify an earliest fill-by date. Patients would still need to make monthly trips to the pharmacy, but they could forgo monthly visits to the doctor. Dr. Peters thought this was an excellent compromise and actively lobbied for MPG members to write the DEA in support of the measure. This sort of lobbying work is a prime example of the translative negotiation that occurs over clinical practice and directly influences the patient, disease, and clinical ontologies staged.

While the insurance industry and the DEA wield immense power over the practice of pain medicine, no two entities in the American medical landscape are more influential than the FDA and the pharmaceutical industry. When it comes to pharmacological practice, the articulated work of these entities has broad and sweeping effects on medical practice, from the availability of certain drugs to control over future directions in research. The pharmaceutical industry is one of the primary funding mechanisms for biomedical research. But individual corporations cannot receive a return on investment without FDA approval. To return to the earlier metaphor, the pharmaceutical industry writes the label and the FDA approves it, enforcing the discursive regulation the label enacts. The multibillion-dollar pharmaceutical industry produces numerous new drugs for which they seek FDA approval. Subsequently, the FDA has to prioritize the order of approval review. However, as would be expected, that prioritization can be a very political process. During a presentation by a pharmaceutical representative/expert in chronic constipation, Dr. Gonsales describes some of these problems:

> There are going to be some very nice products—theoretically. In that "theoretical" is a wasteland of lots of dead products, of products that never quite make it. Now here's the problem: this [constipation] is not an area the FDA thinks is important. These patients aren't going to die. They don't have AIDS. They don't have cancer. They don't have heart disease. So they've got to fill every stringent criteria the FDA puts forward with no fluctuation. There's no fluctuation whatsoever. I need someone on the FDA to be constipated. Then we'll get a little play. Pain would help us there. (MPG Journal Club, November 2007)

According to Dr. Gonsales, issues like chronic constipation and pain management that do not have a high media profile or mortality rate do not receive as much FDA attention. Without these FDA approvals, practitioners cannot offer novel interventions.

The force of FDA regulations even exerts itself on the informal gatherings of the MPG. As we mentioned earlier, MPG discourse is made possible by subsidies from pharmaceutical companies. In exchange for an opportunity to present research on the efficacy of their products, pharmaceutical corporations fund MPG meetings. However, FDA regulations stipulate that pharmaceutical representatives cannot discuss uses for a given drug that have not been officially approved by the FDA. During one presentation, Dr. Gonsales was forced to defer all off-label discussion to the informal Q&A at the end of the talk:

As you know the government—Big Brother's out there listening—this is a pharmaceuticals-sponsored discussion. So I can only talk initially about the FDA-approved indications for the treatment of chronic constipation. But I can tell you I'll be happy to talk to you about your questions. (MPG Journal Club, November 2007)

The representational practices of the MPG exists in a professional space dominated by the recent medical trend toward EBM and by the influence of regulatory agencies such as the FDA and the DEA and the regularizing influence of the insurance industry. As members of the MPG explore the evidential-translative stasis and the question of who has jurisdiction over the definition of pain, the legitimacy of subjective clinical evidence, and the authorization and allocation of practical treatment, they grapple with an additional practical-translative stasis grounded in institutional obstacles to the nonmodern pain ontology. In sum, all of these conflicting regulatory structures form a stasis over who will get to decide which treatment the patient receives—the MPG member, the clinic owner, the insurance company, the FDA, or the DEA?

Reflections on Stases and Calibration

Most of the stases that are activated by MPG members to explore a nonmodern ontology on pain appear in the informal, "off-label" portion of MPG meetings, when members could step outside their disciplinary restrictions and work at ontological calibration. As the MPG president noted to the membership at one meeting, "None of us individually own pain, and yet we all own pain. We need each other's insights and perspectives to get a fuller picture of pain and how to treat patients" (MPG Journal Club, February 2008). One of the best examples of off-label discussion enlisting multidisciplinarity comes from a December 2006 presentation by a pain management physician who researched the importance of restorative sleep. Dr. Steele's presentation began by specifically acknowledging the strengths of various disciplines and inviting them into dialogue:

I love my surgical friends who *can* very effectively treat physical pain. You know, bad disc, bad nerve, bad blood vessels . . . whatever the case. Thank you for coming tonight. But . . . that's physical pain. It's not that simple. I'm gonna use the word emotional pain, psychological pain. Any psychologists here?

Good! Anxiety, MRI, a little claustrophobia, what are the chances of getting a good MRI? That would be zero. Because you're gonna panic and you're going to leave. What if your wife left you? What if you got beat up by your father? There's emotional pain that's real. Physical abuse doesn't go away with a pill. (MPG Journal Club, December 2006)

These off-label discussions inadvertently replicated the logic of stasis theory. Stasis theory is not only a method for identifying the points of departure grounding particular debates, but also a process designed to help foster more coordinated discourse. As Prelli (2005) concludes in his discussion of stasis, no method will reduce controversy unless disputants "acknowledge the potential value of perspectival diversity" (p. 327). And Cicero (1949) argued that sometimes a stasis dispute necessitates the suspension of argument and the engagement of metadiscourse to determine the new stasis from which future argument will derive:

> The controversy about a definition arises when there is agreement as to the fact and the question is by what word that which has been done is to be described. In this case there must be a dispute about the definition, because there is no agreement about the essential point, not because the fact is not certain, but because the deed appears differently to different people, and for that reason different people describe it in different terms. Therefore in cases of this kind the matter must be defined in words and briefly described. (*De Inventione* 1.8.11–12)

During their off-label discussions, members of the MPG work to understand the language and position of other members. At one point, Dr. Bennetti celebrates a recent presentation with which he had greatly disagreed: "We are all in a silo. One of the best [recent presenters] was talking about spinal cord stimulators, and I love the way he thinks. . . . He presented his stuff and it was very good. You learn something. It breaks down those barriers" (MPG Journal Club, May 2008). Or as physician's assistant Hamlyn reflects in a follow-up interview, "I think that sometimes there's a lack of respect among the various disciplines, and some close-mindedness. . . . I think that may be one reason why some of the pain specialists in the community—the physicians, MDs—are less in attendance" (Hamlyn, ethnographic interview).

When individual members of the MPG were asked to discuss their work with what I could call ontological calibration, they were uniformly laudatory. They talk of learning to see pain as an assemblage of puzzle pieces or mosaic tiles. And they comment that the ongoing dialogue has made them understand pain as a more complex phenomenon that supersedes any single discipline. The comments of Dr. Bennetti during an interview are representative of the group's members:

> It creates a fuller picture of what pain is. You appreciate the complexity of the suffering as it relates to the patient's whole world. The complex pharmacology, the social interactions . . . it's kind of hard to describe. It's not an easy thing. Everybody's got a knowledge base that they can give you. (Bennetti, ethnographic interview)

And though my ontological account of this success is different from Bennetti's perspectival account, his words still reinforce the notion of off-label static discourse as a mode of cross-ontological calibration.

The combination of Mol's multiple ontologies with functional stasis analysis allows us to understand the processes through which discursive transformation begins and through which the MPG establishes a nascent nonmodern ontology. For rhetorical-ontological inquiry more broadly, this chapter suggests that functional stasis theory makes visible both the means and the obstacles to ontological calibration that Mol's account model omits. Stasis allows us to understand the concrete and messy work of invention involved in coordinating conflicting ontologies and establishing new ones. And the translative stasis, especially, allows us to explore the material and institutional obstacles to calibration in ways that analyses that elide representational practices do not. As contemporary science grapples with more hybrid phenomena such as pain, PTSD, global warming, and sustainable agriculture, multidisciplinary groups working in these new problem spaces will increasingly struggle to transform scientific discourses. The functional stasis analysis offered here provides one analytic strategy to understand, and possibly foster, this sort of new technoscientific discourse.

CHAPTER FOUR

Neuroimaging Detours

Phantom limb pain is one of the most terrible and fascinating of all clinical pain syndromes.... The phantom limb is usually described as having a tingling feeling and a definite shape that resembles the real limb before amputation. It is reported to move through space in much the same way as the normal limb would move when the person walks, sits down, or stretches out on a bed. At first, the phantom limb feels perfectly normal in size and shape — so much so that the amputee may reach out for objects with the phantom hand, or try to get out of bed by stepping on to the floor with the phantom leg. As time passes, however, the phantom limb begins to change shape. The arm or leg becomes less distinct and may fade away altogether, so that the phantom hand or foot seems to be hanging in mid-air. Sometimes the limb is slowly "telescoped" into the stump until the only hand or foot remain at the stump tip. —Ronald Melzack, *The Puzzle of Pain*

The link between pain and injury seems so obvious that it is widely believed that pain is always the result of physical damage and that the intensity of pain we feel is proportional to the severity of the injury. In general, this relationship between injury and pain holds true: a pinch of a finger usually produces mild pain, while a door slammed on it is excruciating; a small cut hurts a little, while a laceration can be agonizing. However, there are many instances in which the relationship fails to hold up. For example, some people are born without the ability to feel pain even when they are seriously injured (congenital analgesia), and many of us have injuries such as cuts and bruises without feeling any pain until many minutes or hours later (episodic analgesia). In contrast, there are severe pains that are not associated with any known tissue damage or that persist for years after an injury has apparently healed. Clearly the link between injury and pain is highly variable: injury may occur without pain, and pain without injury. This is the essence of the puzzle of pain. —Ronald Melzack and Patrick Wall, *The Challenge of Pain*

P hantom limb pain, psychosomatic pain, and congenital analgesia: these conditions are cited over and over again at the beginning of academic, medical, and popular treatises devoted to describing the puzzle of pain, the mystery of pain, and the war on pain. Each point to a recurrent and debilitating problem for pain science and management, what Melzack and Wall (1982) dub "the variable link" between pain and injury (p. 3). In

The Puzzle of Pain (1973), just below the subheading "The Puzzle," Melzack notes, "These two kinds of cases—the inability to feel pain in spite
of injury and spontaneous pain in the absence of injurious stimulation—
represent the extremes of pain phenomena" (p. 18). This distinction—
between pain and injury—is a necessary outcropping of the two-world
problem. It is an artifact of the separation between mind and body, and
it further results in a debilitating and unethical state of affairs for pain
patients—a pervasive distrust of so-called subjective patient report. In
modernist pain science and medicine, injury is of the body and pain is
of the mind—a division reinforced by a whole host of studies exploring
and documenting the division between injury and pain. Phantom limb pain,
psychosomatic pain, and congenital analgesia are just the beginning. The
manifest efficacy of placebos (Turner, Deyo, Loeser, Von Korff & Fordyce,
1994), the differential pain reports for the same pain stimuli among different
cultural groups (Zatzick & Dimsdale, 1990), and the lower pain thresholds
of redheads (Liem, Joiner, Tsueda & Sessler, 2005) all serve as recurrent
reminders to the medical community that injury and pain are separate and
only occasionally related phenomena.

If that were the end of it, we would have a two-world problem, but
not necessarily an ethical problem. Unfortunately, under the dominant
biomechanical empirical-discursive ontology staged by EBM, the body
wins. The body is the authentic locus of disease, and the mind is confused,
crazy, or simply lying. So pervasive is the lack of trust in patient report
(as confusion, insanity, or malingering) that it is a mainstay of popular
representations of medicine. Indeed, anyone familiar with the 2004–12
hit Fox television series *House M.D.* will recognize the ubiquity of these
views in the recurrent mantra of the series' antihero, Dr. Gregory House:
"Everybody lies." If this were merely a plot device, it would not be so
bad; but the practices of EBM stage an ontology that routinely enforces
the boundary between "subjective patient report" and "objective clinical
findings" (see Shim & Williams, 1983; Ophir, Gross-Isseroff, Lancet &
Maarshak, 1986; Shulman et al., 2006; Shir & Fitzcharles, 2009; Harden,
2010). Correspondingly, scholarship in medical humanities is full of accounts of the marginalization of patient voices and experience, especially
when it comes to ailments perceived to be located in the mind (Anderson,
1996; Resnik, Rehm & Minard, 2001; Graham, 2009, 2011).

This situation provides another opportunity to investigate both the effects of the two-world problem in pain medicine and also another form
of cross-ontological calibration, one I call calibration by detour (CBD).

CBD, as the name suggests, takes on the notion of detour and enlistment from Latour's work on actor-network theory. In *Pandora's Hope* (1999), Latour offers a model of agentive articulation where agents (or programs of action) are unable to accomplish their goal(s) on their own, so they must detour through another agent or program of action in order to accomplish a combined set of goals. In short, CBD describes the rhetorical-ontological processes whereby an interruption in a program of action (in this case, a marginalized ontology) is circumvented by detouring through and enlisting a more authoritative ontology. Specifically, this chapter will investigate efforts by the medical community at large—and pain management specialists in particular—to link subjective patient report to the objective findings of neuroimaging.

In so doing, I investigate two phases of CBD. First, I begin this chapter by exploring the overt discursive process whereby subjective patient report is calibrated to neuroimaging in the MPG. Second, I take my own detour through historical processes whereby neuroimaging is authorized as a powerful point of detour. As part of this historical analysis, this chapter will document process of CBD via *trope shifting*, my term from the discursive dimension of Latourian detour and enrollment. Ultimately, my excavation of CBD in contemporary pain medicine and the history of medical imaging both adds to my growing typology of rhetorical-ontological moves and also points toward the ethical issues that arise from the two-world's creation of the problem of subjective patient report. Finally, I will close this chapter with a return to pain and a brief reflection on the problem of "neuroimperialism" for patient representation.

From "Adding Up" to Calibration by Detour

As mentioned above, the problem of the disjunct between patient subjective report and clinical observations is a recurrent issue in pain medicine. Indeed, it is confronted regularly and directly in the MPG discourse on a variety of conditions. For example, as part of an article summary presentation, an MPG presenter addresses one of the methodological "weaknesses" in the study under discussion:

> I thought the subjective bias was one of the problems, because pain perception is very different from one person to the next. That's something that's hard to overcome, because there's no way for us to find an objective way to assess pain.

Compliance can also be a problem, because we don't know if the patient is taking their medication. (MPG Journal Club, March 2007)

Here the results of the study are presented as suspect because the evidence for disease and improvement came from patient report and not
objective clinical evidence such as blood tests or physical examination.
Despite the recurrent discomfort with subjective patient report, the lack
of available clinical tests makes it a primary source of evidence in pain
science and management.

Mol's work (2002) on adding up and calibration is instructive here,
as her analyses of these processes focus primarily on the problems that
arise when subjective patient report conflicts with diagnostic evidence.
In chapter 2, I discussed Mol's exploration of adding up as a process in
which conflicting findings could be adjudicated in a scorekeeping fashion.
However, the power of objective clinical findings over subjective patient
report challenges the possibility of adding up. As Mol notes, "A hierarchy
between subjective 'complaints' and objectifying 'laboratory findings' is
institutionalized in the very routine that says that all patients with clinical
disease go to the lab before further therapeutic measures are considered"
(2002, p. 63). Although Mol makes some space for the use of adding up
when it comes to conflicting patient report and clinical findings, the institutional hierarchy that subordinates patient complaints to laboratory
data makes adding up in such cases a highly fraught endeavor. How much
patient report does it take to balance out laboratory data? There's no
clear answer to this question, but whatever the number, it is certainly not
a one-to-one ratio. Patient report must be so overwhelmingly powerful
that it counterbalances the objective.

With Mol's adding up largely off the table, one option is the jurisdictional calibration discussed in the previous chapter. Indeed, Dr. Boysen's
lament over the lack of a "pain-o-meter" and the surrounding discussion of this evidential-translative stasis serves as primary exemplar for
this mode of calibration. Pain clinicians can make overt arguments for
the authority of subjective patient report. For example, Dr. Michelson,
the phenomenologist of suffering and orthopedist from the AAPM, gave
an impassioned defense of subjective patient report during our interview:

I think there's great confusion in medical practice about the definition of pain
and suffering. Traditionally, physicians see "suffering" as the affective experience of pain, which can't be true if you understand [that] the subjectivity of

something means you can't measure it, just as you can't measure pain. The subjectivity makes it immune to validation, and immune to objective measurement. There are people who've tried to measure pain and suffering, but one of the first things those concerned will admit [is] there's no algometer, no dial on somebody's forehead. As long as you can't read it out, you have to rely on the patient's report. A lot of physicians don't trust patients. They think that subjective reports are inherently unreliable, untrustworthy. In that perception of untrustworthiness, they demean the experience of pain and suffering. (Michelson, ethnographic interview)

However, when confronted with the power of EBM's empirical-discursive ontology and its staging of the body over the mind, the objective over the subjective, arguments like these do not always carry the day, even within the MPG. Indeed, the passage on methodological weaknesses above is a primary example of this. Similarly, in one question-and-answer session, interventional anesthesiologist Dr. Bennetti calibrates patient report to functional evidence, and in so doing dismisses the validity of patient report:

AUDIENCE MEMBER: Have you had patients where you have had good results, but they walk in saying, "Oh, my pain is still 10"?

DR. BENNETTI: Yeah. Both your points are well taken. I think we all see that in our practice. Psychological gain—or maybe that just speaks to the weakness of the visual analog scale as to how well it can really assess pain. That's why I look at—when I talk about spinal cord stimulation with patients—the case presentations came out the way they were or the way they are, but I tend to do a spinal cord stimulator, and then I'll think about a[n intrathecal] pump if I [could do anything] because I think a stimulator is a fantastic modality. It's reversible. It gives us great information about the anatomy. The pump is— hell, there's nothing more to do now. It's narcotic drug management, and we're avoiding side effects. Those are always those things, but I look at functioning. Look at activities. Even if they report a pain score of 10 out of 10—"What'd you do the other day?" "I walked around [the] lake." Oh, well, that's a different thing when they were unable to go through the parking lot at [the] lake without having pain. (MPG Journal Club, January 2006)

Here, even with the most nonmodern of pain management clinicians, the conflict between patient report (as measured by the visual analog scale) and functional assessments is rendered as a failure of the inventory, a

rejection of patient report. Given the challenges of adding up or translative calibration, another option is required. And as mentioned above, this
option is frequently CBD via neuroimaging.

Within the MPG, neuroimaging as an example of CBD is most often
invoked in regard to marginalized diseases and therapies. In the first case,
fibromyalgia syndrome (FMS) and migraines—two illnesses that dispro-
portionately afflict women and are too often construed as mental illness
(Segal, 2005a; Graham, 2009, 2011) are warranted by detour through neuroimaging. In short, the argument goes: we are told we can't trust these
women's reports of pain, but we can trust neuroimaging data showing
the pain they feel. The following is a passage from a popular press interview with Dr. Muhammad Yunus, a leading FMS researcher. It amplifies
the processes of detouring around the lack of trust in patient report and
through neuroimaging.

> Until recently, doctors didn't believe fibromyalgia pain was real. They thought
> it was "all in the heads" of sufferers, who happened to be mainly women. When
> Dr. Muhammad Yunus of the University of Illinois began studying it in 1977,
> colleagues warned him, "You'll ruin your career. *These women are just crazy.*"
> But the fact that doctors couldn't find a cause or a cure for some 6 million suf-
> ferers didn't mean that the pain wasn't there. *In the past few years scientists
> have used powerful brain scans to provide proof that it is.* Researchers have now
> pinpointed genetic variations that may play a role, and companies are racing
> to provide effective drugs. "It's a new day in fibromyalgia," says Dr. Andrew
> Holman, a Seattle rheumatologist who's testing promising new pills. "We're
> starting to win the battle." (Underwood, 2003, p. 53, emphasis added)

Similarly, psychotherapy and placebo therapy are warranted as efficacious through neuroimaging studies. Patients may say they feel better
after psychotherapy or placebo therapy, but doctors now *know* they feel
better because of neuroimaging.

In the following passage, MPG psychologist Dr. Landau detours
through neuroimaging—in this case functional magnetic resonance imaging (fMRI)—to buttress the practices of placebo therapy:

> The interesting thing on this study was that there was a high variability in who
> responded to placebo. Only eight of the twenty-four on this study showed the
> placebo effect. Later on, they will show that you can raise that number just
> short of placebo there. The interesting thing with the milder shock there wasn't
> as much placebo as with the more severe shot, which, again, this raises more

questions than answers. The interesting thing is when people reported placebo they had less pain. They also showed reduction in the fMRI in the pain centers with placebos. The findings were significant at the .005 level. So somehow placebo changes what happens in the brain. It is not just that they want to do it to please us. Where they found a strong correlation is between reported placebo effects and prefrontal activation that was related to generating and maintaining expectations. Somehow that placebo is related to expectations. We don't know exactly how. We just know that that is what lit it up. (MPG Journal Club, February 2005)

Each of these cases functions as a form of detour and enrollment. The clinical practices of pain management that stage the semiotic pain ontology are interrupted by the empirical-discursive rejection of "subjective patient report." Clinicians and researchers then detour through neuroimaging in order to calibrate the semiotic ontology to the empirical-discursive and in so doing legitimize the practices that stage the semiotic ontology in cases of marginalized diseases.

But what makes CBD work? Obviously, not all detours would be equally effective. If Dr. Landau wanted to warrant subjective patient report and placebo therapy by detouring through acupuncture, I'd wager she'd have considerably less rhetorical success. So, clearly, something about the neuroimager makes it an especially powerful calibrating tool. As many (including myself) have argued, the power of neuroimaging as a detour agent arises from its status as black box (Dumit, 2004; Wisberg, Keil, Goodstein, Rawson & Gray, 2008; Graham, 2009; Jack & Appelbaum, 2010; Brown & Murphy, 2010). The authorization and legitimization of a new technology is generally known, in the language of Latour (1987), as "black boxing"—the process whereby the complexities of a technology are elided and through which the technology is authorized. Latour traces the metaphor of the black box to cybernetics (pp. 3–4). Cyberneticists routinely deal with highly complex scalable computer systems. Sometimes the density of articulations (lines of connections and relationships) in cybernetics subsystems are so complex that the technical details are not needed in order to solve the current (higher-level) problem. So cyberneticists draw a black box around the subsystem and merely address it in terms of input and output. But effective black boxing is not just about the elision of complexity in one moment or context. As Latour (1987) notes, black boxing only becomes more powerful when distributed through time and space: "The black box moves in space and becomes durable in time only through the actions of many people; if there is no one to take it up, it stops and falls apart however many people may have taken it up however long before" (p. 137). The more people who elide the complexity and authorize the technology, the more authority the technology has garnered, thus making it a prime site for detour.

This black boxing of neuroimaging is pervasive and evident in the MPG and popular press extracts above. In none of the above passages were the vagaries of neuroimaging explored. Indeed, "brain scan" is frequently a synecdoche for all neuroimaging technologies in MPG and broader medical discourse. Its use elides an entire pantheon of neuroimaging technologies, including (1) computed axial tomography (CAT/CT), (2) magnetic resonance imaging (MRI), (3) positron emission topography (PET), (4) single photon emission computed tomography (SPECT), and (4) functional magnetic resonances imaging (fMRI). To further complicate matters, each of these is a technology in the abstract sense. Any given device may be manufactured by Philips, GE Health, ROSATOM, or any one of another dozen companies. And each individual company often has an entire line of imaging devices with different brands and models. All of this complexity and multiplicity makes it very difficult to go about the task of identifying how any given technology became a primary tool for CBD.

Nevertheless, there is a certain consistency across these devices. All broadly fall under the category of nuclear imaging technologies. All will typically be found in hospital departments of radiology and used primarily for diagnostic imaging. As such, there is enough consistency to make my inquiry possible. In the sections that follow, my excavation of neuroimaging's utility as a detour site will focus on a detour through X-ray imaging, CT, and PET. In so doing, I propose to unpack the black box of neuroimaging. Of course, unpacking black boxes—that is, identifying the constituent articulations and elided complexities of a given assemblage— has become a routine form of scholarship in STS and rhetorical studies. Indeed, numerous studies (including those listed above) have been devoted to unpacking the black boxes of neuroimaging technologies. In adding to this scholarship, I propose using a different method, one that also exemplifies the rhetorical-ontological processes of CBD.

A Detour on Detours

Medical anthropologist Dumit's (2004) *Picturing Personhood: Brain Scans and Biomedical Identity* is one of the most well-known unpackings of the neuroimaging black box. Dumit's analysis of PET provides a two-part unpacking. In the first place, he details how the complexity of the PET process is elided by the photographic interpretation of neuroimaging technologies. He also traces the way PET images were rather quickly authorized to "speak" in U.S. courts of law through analogous reference to X-ray technologies. In the first unpacking, Dumit argues that despite the discourse that suggests PET scans "take pictures" of the inside of the body, what they actually do is allow physicians to trace the flow of important bodily chemicals such as blood or oxygen. PET-based neuroimaging operates under the assumption that if more blood or oxygen is going to one part of the brain than another, then that part of the brain is being used more by the patient. This is why this technology is often referred to as "functional imaging"—it images not physical structures (anatomy) but bodily functions (physiology). The development of these images involves a complex, multipart process—each step replete with a variety of scientific, technological, and rhetorical decisions. PET image generation requires several steps:

1. The injection of the patient with a "marker" chemical. These markers (of which there are many available) have a particular chemical makeup that allows them to bond with the bodily chemical that the physician wants to trace (for example, blood or oxygen). The markers emit positron radiation (hence the name PET), which is used to track the flow of the marked chemicals. The released positrons (aka antielectrons) collide with electrons already in the body. This collision produces gamma radiation that can be detected by the PET scanning device.
2. The scanning device uses highly complicated mathematics to trace the trajectory of each gamma ray back to its origin, and after assimilating all of the data from each gamma ray, the device creates a mathematical representation of a "slice" of the patient's brain.
3. The data produced by the scanning device is filtered through a software application designed to produce a graphical representation of the data. The data is represented by one of many available predetermined color schemes, each designed for different purposes. Through this process, a brain scan—a four-dimensional representation of the function of a cross-section of the brain—is produced.

Nevertheless, as Dumit explains, despite the complexity of the neuroimaging, "most contemporary understandings of the [PET or] CT scan assume it to unproblematically represent the structure of the brain" (p. 117). This is an assumption that elides the many methodological decisions involved in developing a particular PET scan. PET representations are influenced and changed by (1) the choice of radioisotope, (2) the algorithm chosen for processing the gamma-ray scatter, and (3) the choice of representing color scheme. Essentially, the same brain, scanned at the same time, could be used to generate thousands of different images. As such, a high level of radiological literacy is required to properly interpret a neuroimaging.

While this mode of unpacking is very useful in problematizing the simple conceits that surround neuroimaging, it is less helpful in identifying how neuroimaging became an eligible site for CBD. A more productive line of inquiry comes from Dumit's analysis of the acceptance of neuroimaging testimony in courts of law. In this later analysis, he traces arguments for the use of CT scans in the trial of John Hinckley for the attempted assassination of Ronald Reagan. Hinckley's attorney sought permission from the court to use CT scans to demonstrate the defendant's insanity and thus lack of culpability for his actions. Eventually, the judge ruled in the defense's favor and allowed the images. What Dumit documents in his second unpacking is how the history of medical imaging in U.S. law courts paved the way for this decision. This historiographic work begins with an interrogation of an 1896 decision to allow X-ray images as evidence in the courtroom. Dumit's analysis argues that X-rays were ultimately admitted due to a "sophisticated deferral" wherein the new technology was fused into the discourses of cartography and photography (p. 114). As evidence for this claim, Dumit provides the following passage from the judge's decision:

> We [the court] have nothing to do or say as to what [the radiographs] purport to represent; that will, without doubt, be explained by eminent surgeons. These exhibits are only pictures or maps, to be used in explanation of a present condition, and therefore secondary evidence and not primary. (*Smith v. Grant*, 1896, as cited in Dumit, 2004, p. 114)

Moving forward from this point, Dumit explores how newer imaging technologies (CT, PET) are linked to X-rays in much the same sort of sophisticated deferral in which X-rays were linked to photography and cartography. In short, Dumit explains how black boxes can be borrowed and how that process of borrowing can accelerate the process of black boxing for novel technologies.

While Dumit offers a compelling account of the black boxing of neuroimaging in courts of law, I am more interested in how that technology became black boxed within medical science. As noted above, Latour argues clearly that time and distance contribute significantly to black boxing. The farther away one gets from the source of innovation (temporally or contextually), the more easily the complexity of novel technology is elided. Jurisprudential practices are fairly removed from the sciences of diagnostic imaging. As such, it should come as no surprise how quickly imaging technologies were black boxed and accepted. (Although, as the following analysis helps to indicate, I think Dumit may have overstated the speed of acceptance for X-rays in 1896.) Subsequently, in the next section I will begin a historical unpacking of the imaging technologies that focuses on the sites of development for these technologies rather than the sites of appropriation and extension.

Trope Shifting and Articulation

Typical approaches to the study of black boxes follow the models of Dumit and Latour—that is, they are principally concerned with identification and unpacking. As such, the study of black boxes often appears synchronic and structuralist—the identified material-semiotic node has power; here's why. However, such an orientation does not allow for a thorough appreciation of CBD, the diachronic process of black-box formation. A historical tracing of the development of a black-boxed technology provides an opportunity to understand both the nature of its power and the mechanisms of articulation that led to the establishment of the black box in the first place. The following section investigates the historical emergence of the now black-boxed colocation of nuclear medical technologies (eventually PET and fMRI) and photography. In Latourian terms, this is a process of articulation and enrollment. In Mol's vernacular, black boxing is a process of calibration. Either theoretical overlay helps an analyst understand the unification of technologies that is the colocation of nuclear medicine and photography. However, neither provides the analyst with a vocabulary for understanding the rhetorical dimension that coordinates with the ontological; thus, I join the two under the umbrella of CBD.

In order to help establish a truly hybrid rhetorical-ontological accounting of black boxing in action, I turn to the concept of "trope shifting." Trope shifting is my term for a change in language patterns I have identified as part of the black boxing of nuclear medicine qua photography.

That is, as the historical patterns of action and discourse that surround the nuclear medicine/photography coupling change and co-articulate, the tropic form of that relationship changes. Typically, in rhetorical studies, tropic analysis takes the form of investigating the rationale behind or the effects of the author's strategic deployment of specific tropes and figures. How does the "city on a hill" metaphor inspire patriotism among conservative American audiences? How does Stephen Colbert's use of irony expose the excesses of cable news punditry? In critical-cultural rhetorical studies and STS, the use of tropic analysis is more structural. Evelyn Fox Keller interrogates the cultural effects of the blueprint and code metaphors used by biologists to describe DNA. Similarly, Donna Haraway (1997) excavates the salvationist overtones of contemporary technological discourse. In each of these modes of inquiry, the investigation of tropes centers on the introduction of a figure of speech into discourse and its effects. In the case of traditional rhetorical studies, the focus is on the effects wrought by an individual rhetor's strategic deployment of a trope in a specific context. In critical-cultural rhetorics and STS, the investigations center around how certain figures of speech are complicit in maintaining hegemonic structures. Within either approach, a great deal of agency is invested in the metaphor itself. Certainly it is the displaced agency of either the rhetor in the first case or the structure in the second, but the power of the metaphor is central to the analysis in both. Of course, I recognize the power of tropes and figures over audiences, cultures, practices, and ontologies. Indeed, following Dumit and others, I argue that the figurative relationship between medical imaging and photography is part of why medical imaging has so much power—and this becomes a valuable resource for CBD.

At its core, a figure of speech is a linguistic articulation. I. A. Richards (1936) famously defines the metaphor quite technically as the joining of a "vehicle" and a "tenor" (p. 96), the vehicle being that idea or object from which properties are borrowed. So in the cases of the world being a stage or love being a rose, the stage and the rose are vehicles and the world and love are tenors. In introducing this technical lexicon for metaphor criticism, Richards works to distance the study of metaphors from a whole host of then-traditional assumptions, including (1) the need for metaphors to be an intentional stylistic decision rather than a fundamental facet of language, (2) the understanding of metaphor as a mere ornament, (3) the unteachability of metaphor, and (4) the a priori understanding of metaphors as sense extensions based in resemblance. Richards's approach to metaphor is observational and descriptive. He entreats readers not to declare, in advance, the nature and effects of metaphor, but rather to watch them unfold in language and then draw conclusions:

> Let us consider more closely what happens in the mind when we put together—in a sudden and striking fashion—two things belonging to very different orders of experience. The most important happening—in addition to a general confused reverberation and strain—are the mind's efforts to connect them. The mind is a connecting organ, it works only by connecting and it can connect any two things in an indefinitely large number of different ways. Which of these it chooses is settled by reference to some larger whole or aim. (pp. 124–125)

Richards goes on to explore a range of possible responses to a series of vehicle-tenor couplings. While the details of his analysis are beyond the scope of the present discussion, it's critical to note that he makes room for very complicated modes of relationship between a vehicle and a tenor, including relationships of antithesis. Thus, I would argue that Richards is offering us a propositional theory of metaphor. That is, when a rhetor deploys a vehicle-tenor coupling, it is a proposal of resemblance. The linguistic thrift of metaphors relies on the audience to supply the nature of the vehicle-tenor relationship. As such, a metaphor-as-proposition makes room for the possibility of rejection. Indeed, we have all been party to conversations wherein one of the discussants declares a proposed metaphor inappropriate. Such a declaration is typically an assertion that the vehicle does not adequately resemble the tenor. Following Richards, my trope-shifting analysis takes an untheorized vehicle-tenor coupling as its center. However, rather than explore the cognitive processes of relationship in an individual mind, my analysis focuses on what forms of relationship the historical and practical contexts operationalize. Whereas Richards describes the selection of relationships as a result of "reference to some larger whole or aim" of the individual, I understand the selection of relationships to be the result of a reference to the larger whole of the ontology or emergent metaphysics. That is, the arrangements or articulations that surround the use of a particular vehicle-tenor coupling authorize certain relationships.

And to this analysis, I add Burke's more nuanced lexicon of tropic analysis. In his discourse on the four master tropes, Burke (1969) suggests that metaphors, metonymies, and synecdoches are overlapping forms. He further argues that each of these terms can be reinterpreted as perspective, reduction, and representation, respectively. A metaphor challenges the audience to see one thing in terms of another. A metonymy reduces an intangible idea to the perspective of a tangible one. A synecdoche represents a whole by reducing it to the perspective of one of its parts. Following this reinterpretation, we can understand the relationship between these three tropes to be hierarchical. Synecdoche is a form of metonymy, and both are forms of metaphor. Rereading Burke and Richards through each other, I understand Burke's reinterpretation as a specification of the modes of relationship available in a given vehicle-tenor coupling:

- A *metaphor* is a proposal to the audience to view a tenor in terms of a vehicle. As a proposal, it is more open to contestation and rejection.
- A given metaphor is said to be a *metonymy* when the possibilities of relationship are more circumscribed. Something about the context (the surrounding articulations) limits the possibilities for contestation. There is said to be an a priori logical relationship between the vehicle and the tenor, such that one can be reduced to the other. Thus, there is a tighter fit between the vehicle and the tenor.
- Similarly, where the possible relationships (articulations) between a vehicle and a tenor are even further circumscribed (whole/part, sign/signified, container/contained, and so on), the metaphor in question is said to be a *synecdoche*. The resemblance between the vehicle and the tenor is correspondingly more powerful still.

Following these definitions, we can understand a progressive relationship between metaphor, metonymy, and synecdoche. A historical transition from one to the next is a trope shift, and that shift represents a change in the audience's understanding of the relationships (articulations) between the vehicle and tenor. Thus, we have a stronger and more powerful relationship between the two. And it is here that we can see the special utility of trope shifting in exploring the historical establishment of a black box and CBD. The power and authority of black boxes is defined by their self-effacing density of articulations. This density of articulations is the context in which the fit between the vehicle and the tenor is determined. As such, I take, as the center of my analysis, the linguistic entanglements of medical imaging and photography. What I will document is not so much the strategic deployment of those entanglements but how the evolving contexts of both medical imaging and photography serve to change the nature of those entanglements. Specifically, as I trace the history of nuclear medical diagnostics, I note a shift from metaphor, to metonymy, to synecdoche. That is, the tightness of the relationship between the vehicle and tenor increases as the technological imbroglio is black boxed (arranged or articulated). This process is the essence of CBD.

Metaphor

As Dumit recognized, this history of diagnostic X-ray technology is intimately tied up with photography. Wilhelm Röntgen, who is widely credited with the discovery of X-rays, also created the first X-ray image by asking his wife to place her hand between an X-ray emitter and photographic plates. And indeed, as early as 1896 Arthur Brunel Chatwood published a book titled *The New Photography* that included a lengthy section on X-rays in addition to color, psychic, and spirit photography. Despite these early articulations of X-ray and photographic technology, the contemporary idea of X-ray imaging as photographic technology did not immediately take root, at least not in the medical community. As my gloss of Richards would put it, the proposed metaphor of medical imaging as photography was contested. A primary indicator of this contestation can be found in the proliferation of contested terminology used to refer to these "images": X-ray photograph, shadowgraph, skiagraph, skiagram, electrograph, radiogram, röntogenogram, radiograph, and so on. Indeed, in the following excerpt from the correspondence section of the *British Medical Journal* (1897), Charles H. Wade argues that X-ray imaging should be dubbed *electography* as opposed to any of the other possible names. In so doing, Wade demonstrates the propositional (and therefore open to contestation) nature of the relationship between X-ray imaging and photograph:

> Wanted, a Name—"Electrography."
>
> SIR,—In common with most of those who have evinced a permanent interest in the remarkable discoveries of Professor Roentgen in connection with the x ray phenemena [*sic*], I have experienced difficulty in finding words suitable for employment under varying conditions, in speaking or writing of the effects resulting from the activity of the rays. The terms so far in use to this end, such as "Roentgen rays," "x rays," "shadowgraph," "skiagraph," "skiagram," etc., leave much to be desired, and it has again and again been lamented that no

generally acceptable terminology, of uniform character, has so far been devised for common use. To meet this want it has occurred to me that the word
"electrography " fulfills the necessary conditions, and that out of it the words
"electrogram," "electrographic," and "electrograph" readily offer themselves
as accurate and expressive. Common agreement has authorised the use of similarly constructed synonyms in the cases of the telegraph, the phonograph, and
in photography; and inasmuch as the X ray pictures are electrically imprinted
productions, they can be said to be "electrograms" in the strictest sense of the
word. Equally also with the other suggested applications of the root term; and
I venture therefore to propose the adoption of names above given as a solution
of a universally-admitted difficulty. (Wade, 1987)

This passage offers important insights into the extent of photography–
medical imaging articulations. As Wade notes, the relationship proposed
between X-rays and photography is no more densely articulated than the
relationship between radiography and telegraphy or radiography and
phonography. In fact, by providing this range of options, Wade's argument
indicates a stronger association between radiography and the inscriptive
suffix (-*graphy*) as opposed to the imaging prefix (*photo*-).

Indeed, I also argue that the passage from *Smith v. Grant* used in Dumit's analysis actually provides additional evidence for the loose articulation between X-ray imaging and photography in the 1890s. The judge's
reticence to offer an opinion as to the nature of the representation is a
key point of evidence. Second, Dumit may be reading the judge's use of
the word *picture* somewhat anachronistically. Although contemporary usage chiefly identifies pictures with photography, this was a relatively recent extension in 1896. The 1828–1884 editions of *Webster's Dictionary*
all identify a picture as the result of drawing or painting. Photography as
a method of making a picture was not added to *Webster's* until 1890, and
only then as the fourth medium following painting, drawing, and engrav-
ing. While this is early enough to make it possible that the author of the
Smith v. Grant opinion had photography in mind when using the word
picture, it is far from definitive.

Additionally, the distance between X-ray technology and photography is maintained in early descriptions of X-ray imaging systems that
separate the X-ray elements from the photographic elements. A survey
of radiography patent applications demonstrates a consistent separation
between the X-ray emission device and the image-capturing technology.
For example, one application filed in 1896 reads, "My invention is an

original apparatus in the nature of an improved lantern for employing the Roentgen or X rays for experimental, demonstrative, or practical purposes. For convenience, by way of reference, I have styled the apparatus a 'radiopticon'" (Easton, 1897). Notice here how the proposed metaphor is *lantern*. X-rays are akin to a light source, not to an imaging device. In fact, the entire application contains only one brief mention of X-ray reception by something that might be what we would now call an imaging device: "The rays are received upon and arrested by a fluorescent screen, and the person or object to be exposed to them is set between it and the lantern." Following the logic of this application, I would argue that at least as of 1896, insofar as X-rays are related to photography, they are the light, the sun, the flashbulb. Another patent application from 1897 describes a procedure whereby stereoscopic images can be produced with X-rays (Thomson, 1897). In this application, it is the X-ray emission mechanism that is elided and the production of what we would anachronistically call 3-D images with photographic plates is explored.

In each of the applications and the countless applications like them, we can see a double separation between X-rays and photography. There is a physical separation; the patient is interposed between the X-ray device and the photographic plates. Additionally, there is a logical separation. X-ray imaging and photography are metaphorical in the propositional sense. The tenor-vehicle coupling is open to contestation and reinterpretation. Although we anachronistically interpret the joining of X-ray and photography as a vehicle-tenor resemblance based in functionality and output, there was clearly a wider range of possible interpretations in the 1890s. X-ray qua light and radiography qua inscription are chief among these.

Metonymy

A relative lack of articulation density between the irradiating device and the photographic technology is maintained in the practices and discourses of successive radiologic devices, at least through the introduction of computerized transverse axial scanning—CAT or CT scans. While the origin of CT may date as far back as 1917, and there is much debate over priority in both history and radiography, the work of Godfrey Hounsfield is largely credited for demonstrating conclusively the value of CT technology (Mould, 1993, p. 92). In his exposition on the need for a new diagnostic investigatory protocol, Hounsfield (1973a) begins by reinscribing X-ray technology in a way that maintains the distinction: "For many years past, X-ray techniques have been developed along the same lines, namely the recording on photographic film of the shadow of the object to be viewed" (p. 1016). This separation is further maintained in his discussion of CT scans:

> The technique to be described divides the head into a series of slices, each being irradiated via its edges; the radiation is confined to the slice and for this reason, unlike conventional X-ray techniques, the information derived from any object within the slice is unaffected by variations in the material on either side of the slice. Data are processed and displayed by digital computer methods. (p. 1016)

In the case of both X-rays and CT scans, praxiographic analysis is instructive. The practices of radiologic imaging (whether via X-ray or CT scan) involve a physical separation between the X-ray emitter and the imaging technology (photographic plates and films or computerized processing). The patient under evaluation is physically placed between the rays and the imager in the case of X-rays, whereas in the case of CT there is a temporal separation. That is, the patient is scanned and then the resulting data is sent to a computer for processing. These practices do not stage an ontology of medical imaging as camera. The distances (physical and/or temporal) do not align with the practices of photography—where, at the time, the imaging device and the film were contained in the very same apparatus. However, the practices of CT scanning are arguably more akin to the photography of the day than X-ray imaging was to its photographic counterpart. As Hounsfield further elaborates, "These are stored in a disc file for processing by a mini computer. A picture is reconstructed from the data by the following method" (1973a, p. 1016). In much the same way as a film camera of the 1970s, where the light ray receptor (lens) and imaging technology (film) are housed in the same physical object (quite often, literally a black box), CT devices would scan patients and record the data to a medium (disc) for further processing. Just as film needed to be developed, the CT data needed to be processed.

This shift in the physicality of radiography from interposed patient to colocated scanning and storage paved the way for a tighter correspondence in the comparative relationship between medical imaging and cameras. Here we have our first trope shift. The proposed metaphor of "X-rays are like cameras" is displaced by a metonymy "CT scanners take pictures." Indeed, the photography/camera metaphor becomes much more apparent in discussions of CT data processing and subsequent image generation.

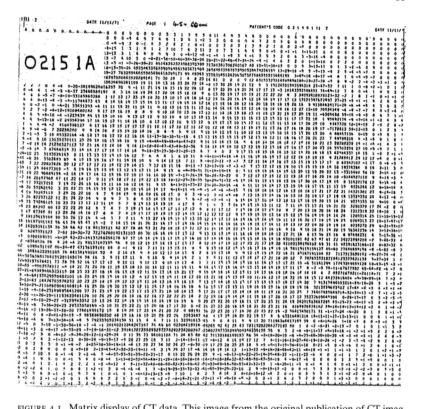

FIGURE 4.1. Matrix display of CT data. This image from the original publication of CT imaging shows an 80 × 80 matrix representing radiation absorption numbers during a brain scan. The use of the matrix as opposed to a more photo-real representation is suggestive of the distance between neuroimaging and photography. Reprinted by permission from Ambrose (1973), figure 17a.

See Hounsfield's description of the bridge between scanning and image generation in his patent abstract:

In apparatus for examining a body by means of X or Y radiation, a two-dimension matrix of elements of the body is exposed to radiation from a number of directions and the transmission of the radiation by a plurality of paths of small cross-sectional area through the body is measured, the directions and numbers of the paths being such that each element of the matrix is intersected by a group of paths which intersect different groups of elements. From these measurements, the absorption or transmission of the individual elements are calculated to produce a cathode ray tube display and/or a photograph. (Houns-field, 1973b)

Here, the patent abstract describes the ways different rates of X-ray ab-sorption by patient tissues are plotted to a matrix of data points. These data points are processed into an image. The tightness of the link between CT and camera is evidenced in Hounsfield's identification of each data point of the matrix as a "picture point": "The picture is built up in the form of an 80 × 80 matrix of picture points to each of which a numeri-cal value is ascribed. Each of these points indicates the value of the ab-sorption coefficient of the corresponding volume of material in the slice" (1973a, p. 1018). Here, the use of *picture* is key. By the 1961 edition of *Webster's Dictionary*, photography is listed as the primary medium of pic-ture making.

While Hounsfield's article focuses primarily on the scanning portion of CT imaging, a companion piece by James Ambrose (1973) clarifies the imagining methodology. Here he provides readers of the *British Journal of Radiology* with the once common matrix image, in which each X-ray absorption value is plotted to its relative location. The resulting matrix of data points hints at a photographic representation of the brain. While more photo-real images were available immediately, the occasional use of the matrix image serves to reinforce the still only metonymic nature of the CT-camera coupling. CT scans are made not by direct imprint on photographic film, but rather by the algorithmic reconstruction of X-ray absorption rates as mapped to a particular patient's physiology. There is clearly something quite similar about the two technologies, but they are not yet understood to be logically identical.

Synecdoche

A significant shift occurs with the next generation of diagnostic devices. An explosion in medical imaging technologies followed closely on the heels of the invention and popularization of CT scans. CT was arguably the first major innovation in medical imaging since the invention of the X-ray in the 1890s. However, articles were published and patents filed for two similarly revolutionary devices within less than a decade of the announcement of CT: nuclear magnetic resonance (NMR) and positron emission transaxial tomography (PETT). NMR and PETT are the earli-est prototypes for what would soon become household names, MRI and

PET, respectively. With the invention and promulgation of NMR and PETT, the trope shifting from metaphor to metonymy to synecdoche becomes complete. Perhaps the most obvious evidence for this comes for the patent titles for successive devices. Wherein X-ray patents were divided into X-ray- or Röntgen-ray-producing devices and photographic devices, the combined CT scanning systems were patented as "radiography" and a "radiation examining apparatus." The initial patents for NMR and PETT identify the former as an "imaging system" and the latter as an "imaging device." While this titular shift might seem minor, I would argue that it provides strong evidence for the emergence of a tacit assumption of a specific logical relationship between medical imaging and photography. CT scanners were diagnostic tools that graphed X-rays. A CT technician could use the device to produce a matrix, a matrix image, a computer display, or a photograph. In contrast, NMR and PETT are understood to be native image producers.

Ter-Pogossian's (1979) PETT patent abstract demonstrates the centrality of the image in positron emission tomography:

> This invention relates to an imaging device for nuclear medicine and, more particularly, to an imaging device which provides a reconstruction of an area under examination by forming tomographic sectional images of the human body under examination subsequent to the administration of radio pharmaceuticals. . . . To facilitate an understanding of the invention, computed axial tomography can be analogized to taking a series of "salami slices" through a patient under examination and utilizing the contents of the slices for image construction. (U.S. Patent No. 4,150,292, issued 1979)

This passage is illustrative in its reference to the proposed metaphor of "salami slices." Here Ter-Pogossian demonstrates his awareness of the pedagogic value of comparing unfamiliar objects to familiar ones. However, he betrays no awareness that "imaging" is metaphorical. Even though Ter-Pogossian is acutely aware of the many details and complexities of tomographic image "reconstruction," he still refers to the product of PETT scanning as simply an "image." This is perhaps all the more interesting given the praxiographic similarity between PETT and CT. While the subatomic physics of PETT is markedly different from CT, that process is invisible—literally outside of the human visual spectrum. In each case, a patient is placed in a scanning device and bombarded with radiation, a matrix of data points is produced, and a visual representation is

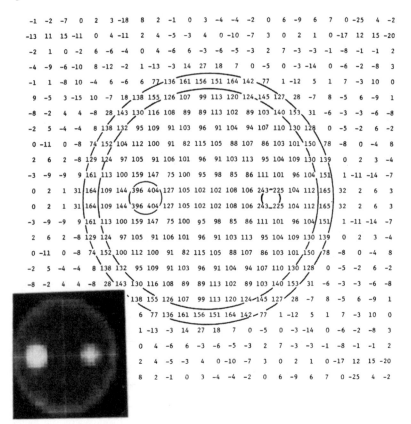

```
 -1  -2  -7   0   2   3 -18   8   2  -1   0   3  -4  -4  -2   0   6  -9   6   7   0 -25   4  -2
-13  11  15 -11   0   4 -11   2   4  -5  -3   4   0 -10  -7   3   0   2   1   0 -17  12  15 -20
 -2   1   0  -2   6  -6  -4   0   4  -6   6  -3  -6  -5  -3   2   7  -3  -3  -1  -8  -1  -1   2
 -4  -9  -6 -10   8 -12  -2   1 -13  -3  14  27  18   7   0  -5   0  -3 -14   0  -6  -2  -8   3
 -1   1  -8  10  -4   6  -6   6  77 136 161 156 151 164 142  77   1 -12   5   1   7  -3  10   0
  9  -5   3 -15  10  -7  18 138 155 126 107  99 113 120 124 145 127  28  -7   8  -5   6  -9   1
 -8  -2   4   4  -8  28 143 130 116 108  89  89 113 102  89 103 140 153  31  -6  -3  -3  -6  -8
 -2   5  -4  -4   8 138 132  95 109  91 103  96  91 104  94 107 110 130 128   0  -5  -2   6  -2
  0 -11   0  -8  74 152 104 112 100  91  82 115 105  88 107  86 103 101 150  78  -8   0  -4   8
  2   6   2  -8 129 124  97 105  91 106 101  96  91 103 113  95 104 109 130 139   0   2   3  -4
 -3  -9  -9   9 161 113 100 159 147  75 100  95  98  85  86 111 101  96 104 151   1 -11 -14  -7
  0   2   1  31 164 109 144 396 404 127 105 102 102 108 106 243 225 104 112 165  32   2   6   3
  0   2   1  31 164 109 144 396 404 127 105 102 102 108 106 243 225 104 112 165  32   2   6   3
 -3  -9  -9   9 161 113 100 159 147  75 100  95  98  85  86 111 101  96 104 151   1 -11 -14  -7
  2   6   2  -8 129 124  97 105  91 106 101  96  91 103 113  95 104 109 130 139   0   2   3  -4
  0 -11   0  -8  74 152 100 112 100  91  82 115 105  88 107  86 103 101 150  78  -8   0  -4   8
 -2   5  -4  -4   8 138 132  95 109  91 103  96  91 104  94 107 110 130 128   0  -5  -2   6  -2
 -8  -2   4   4  -8  28 143 130 116 108  89  89 113 102  89 103 140 153  31  -6  -3  -3  -6  -8
                         138 155 126 107  99 113 120 124 145 127  28  -7   8  -5   6  -9   1
                       6  77 136 161 156 151 164 142  77   1 -12   5   1   7  -3  10   0
                       1 -13  -3  14  27  18   7   0  -5   0  -3 -14   0  -6  -2  -8   3
                       0   4  -6   6  -3  -6  -5  -3   2   7  -3  -3  -1  -8  -1  -1   2
                       2   4  -5  -3   4   0 -10  -7   3   0   2   1   0 -17  12  15 -20
                       8   2  -1   0   3  -4  -4  -2   0   6  -9   6   7   0 -25   4  -2
```

FIGURE 4.2. Matrix and photographic displays of PETT scan. This juxtaposition of matrix display and photographic displays provides additional evidence for the increasingly tight coupling between neuroimaging and photography. Reprinted by permission from Ter-Pogossian, Phelps, Hoffman, and Mullani (1975), figure 5.

reconstructed. Indeed, the initial publication of PETT in *Radiology* even displays a highly similar—although *less* photo-real matrix image (Ter-Pogossian, Phelps, Hoffman & Mullani, 1975). Nevertheless, in the early discourses of CT, data is stored and sent for reconstruction, and, in PETT, images are produced.

Interestingly, although NMR and early MRI devices and systems patents are issued as "imaging devices," the language of the patents is much less image focused than PETT. This may be due to the fact that Hounsfield was issued one of the first NMR patents and his description of the device mirrored the metonymic (as opposed to synecdochic) CT-camera coupling. MRI and fMRI patents maintained a greater distance from the imaging metaphor until the mid-1990s. Fascinatingly, the available data suggests that this shift may have had as much to do with developments in photography as with developments in MRI technology. Indeed, in many ways there was a technological convergence in the history of both photographic and medical imaging, all made possible by microcomputer processing. Thus we have an increasing density of articulations between neuroimaging and photography, articulations that now detour through computer processing.

While there is no smoking gun that firmly demonstrates an interpretive link between digital photography and digital medical imaging, it is clear that they were both undergoing significant technological development around the same time and capturing the popular imagination at about the same rate. Google Ngram, for example, demonstrates a very similar increasing trajectory for the terms "digital photography" and "neuro-imaging" for 1984–2002. Each term undergoes a meteoric rise in use during this time period. Additionally, one can see a similar increase in frequency for each term in a LexisNexis search of major world newspapers. "Neuro-imaging" appears in 3 sources in the 1980s, 47 sources in the 1990s, and 609 sources in the 2000s. Similarly, "digital photography" appears not once in the 1980s, 186 times in the 1990s, and 807 times in the 2000s.

The 1990s simultaneously marks the rise of popular digital photography and a rapid development of neuroimaging technology. The first commercially available digital camera, the Dycam-1, was released in 1990. Around the same time, MRI patents become perfused with the language of "digital imaging." The most interesting and suggestive evidence I could find for the link between MRI and digital photography comes from the 1992 renaming of the medical digital image storage and communications standard. In the 1980s, the growing availability of imaging systems spurred the American College of Radiology to institute a single international standard for imaging data. They partnered with the National Electrical Manufacturers Association to develop this standard, originally called ACR/NEMA 300. However, in 1992, not long after the introduction of the Dycam-1 into consumer markets, ACR/NEMA 300 was renamed digital imaging and communications in medicine, or DICOM. Dean Bidgood, one of the authors of the DICOM standard, told me he doesn't recall whether the rebranding was an intentional homage to the Dycam-1:

> I was a member of Working Group 6, the base standard working group during the time when we were brainstorming about names and logos for the standard. I had been working with other potential user groups outside of diagnostic

radiology for some time at that point and was convinced we needed an open name. The potential user base of DICOM included every entity who used images, waveforms, and image-related data. Other groups needed an inclusive name, to be able to promulgate the standard among their constituencies. Other WG6 members agreed. We needed to change the name significantly, but we also needed to stay as close as possible to the past trajectory, so we would not harmfully destabilize the relationship with our principal stakeholders of that day (ACR and NEMA). It was a fundamental strategic change. But fortunately, the root of the new name was already present in the name of the original standard itself—which, as you said, was the ACR-NEMA Standard. ACR-NEMA Version 2 included a subtitle about digital imaging and communications. So we were able to find a reasonable convergence between the vision of the founding stakeholders and the strategy of the burgeoning new community of stakeholders: the "DICOM" Standard. It was officially the ACR-NEMA Standard for Digital Imaging and Communications in Medicine, Version 3.0. But as we went forward, through various steps, the short form, "DICOM," became the name by which everyone inside and outside of radiology referred to the standard. (Bidgood, personal communication, e-mail, December 11, 2012)

While I was certainly hoping Dr. Bidgood would confirm that the link between DICOM and Dycam-1 was intentional, I nevertheless think that the assonance between the terms serves to demonstrate the zeitgeist of the 1990s and its celebration of all things digital. It is this contextual shift that principally serves to mark the shift from metonymy to synecdoche in the medical imaging/photography coupling. As previously mentioned, the distinction between metonymy and synecdoche is marked by a further circumscription in the possible modes of relationship between the vehicle and the tenor. The perception of not only a logical congruity between medical imaging and photography, but also a close relationship under the umbrella of digital imaging technologies, makes the coupling synecdochic. The culture and audience that appreciates the linguistic coupling must recognize and accept the specific logical relationship.

Black Boxing and Calibration by Detour

Ultimately, tracing this progression from metaphor to metonymy to synecdoche demonstrates a more nuanced relationship between medical imaging and prior technologies such as photography than other imaging histories have offered. (Indeed, this relationship will turn out to play an important role in efforts to ontologize FMS.) The tightness of the fit between the vehicle and the tenor was actually the result of long-term technological developments in both medical imaging and photography. However, it is the very length of this progression that serves to invest in contemporary imaging technologies so much power and the corresponding possibility of CBD. Indeed, as Latour notes, it is the long-term durability of black boxes that renders them so powerful. Similarly, as Dumit suggested in his interrogation of PET, newer imaging technologies are able to more rapidly pass into a black-boxed state through the aforementioned "sophisticated deferral." Thus, successive imaging technologies are metaphorically related to photography and each other in order to operationalize this deferral. This is a prime example of CBD. The relative newness of a recently discovered imaging device constitutes an interruption that is circumvented by tropicly linking the new technology to its forerunners. For example, there is a significant historical, material, and discursive link between PET and X-ray technology. Practical similarities between the two technologies aside, the location of PET within the disciplinary structures and departmental offices of radiology make the PET/X-ray relationship almost a foregone conclusion. In fact, in its original presentation to the scientific community (in the journal *Radiology*), PET was presented as a more sophisticated extension of previous radiological technologies: "positron-emission transaxial tomographic reconstruction permits the visualization of structures which are not ordinarily perceptible with conventional nuclear medicine imaging devices" (Ter-Pogossian, Phelps, Hoffman & Mullani, 1975, p. 96).

Medical discourse also calibrates and authorizes PET by detouring through other black-boxed technologies besides the X-ray and the photograph. The cartography metaphor is prevalent in many articles that discuss the use of PET for functional mapping of the brain (for example, see Roland, 1985, p. 103). In one presentation offered to the MPG on fibromyalgia, the presenter legitimized the PET scan and other similar technologies through reference to the microscope:

Van Leeuwenhoek really did look down through the microscope and he saw cells. He saw it through reflected light. The point is he saw cells and he reconceived himself in the same moment he saw those cells. And he reconceived everything that we know about biological sciences. He described extending and contracting organisms. . . . What is our modern [equivalent]? I call it our "interior multilinearscope." Because it's always something new. It was CT scans, then it was MRIs, then it was PET scans, then it was SPECT scans, and now it's fMRI. . . . But the new interior multilinearscope is fMRI—I think that's about what we're up to. (MPG Journal Club, February 2008)

Indeed, the microscope analogy may well be a common one both for PET and FMS. AAPM speaker and fibromyalgia patient Martinez also invoked the microscopy metaphor during her participant interview with me—recognizing, and questioning, the dominance of ocular centrism in contemporary science:

We're working with a whole new paradigm as medicine moves forward, obviously. If you don't have the technological tools to be able to see something—which is what humans tend to want, is to see something and have it proven over and over again—it's very difficult for science, so to speak, to understand or accept something. . . . My dad was a biologist, and I remember that when I was about six years old, he gave me a microscope for Christmas, and I took the slide with the pond water on it, and all of a sudden I saw all of these creatures living and moving in this little drop of water, which I couldn't have understood or explained or believed in until I had that microscope. [However,] I think it's important that we realize that even though we may not have the tools to understand new things, that human suffering has to come first. If you have something that people are saying over and over again, it makes sense that even though we don't have all the answers or a complete understanding, that you can't just say, "Well, we're going to wait for science to prove it or science to catch up with the technology." (Martinez, ethnographic interview)

When it comes to PET, its invention, subsequent legitimization, and appropriation for medical diagnostics occur at the confluence of multiple deferrals throughout history. Western epistemology's focus on ocular centrism, the invention of microscopy, X-ray technology, X-ray diffraction crystallography, and CT scans all contributed to the changes that resulted in the invention and legitimization of PET, MRI, fMRI and so on.

In order to better account for the two orders of metaphor involved in the historical black boxing of medical imaging technologies, I have provided my own modification of Latour's model of detours and enrollment—what happens when a program of action encounters some form of interruption that prevents it from accomplishing its goal. The result is a detour, Latour's term for when the interrupted program of action aligns itself with

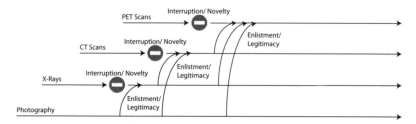

FIGURE 4.3. Multiple enlistments in the neuroimaging black boxing. This modification of Latour's notion of enlistment displays the relationship between various technologies as they
encounter the interruptive force of novelty and work to rapidly circumvent that interruption
through enlisting (taking up) the legitimacy of prior imaging technologies.

another program of action and the two coordinate to accomplish a new
combined goal. I would argue that the calibration of successive medical
imaging technologies was as much about enlistment as it was about detour. The novelty of innovation is its own interruption. It prevents the new
technology from rapidly acquiring legitimacy. The novelty has to wear off
first (temporal distance). However, as Dumit demonstrates in his discussion of PET, novelty can be rapidly elided by deferral, by taking up the
legitimacy of a prior technology. PET did not merely join X-ray in order
to accomplish X-ray goals. It appropriated X-ray legitimacy. It enlisted it.

As figure 4.3 indicates, each enlistment is multiplied. X-rays enlist photography. CT enlists X-rays and photography. And PET undergoes a tri-
ple enlistment where the legitimacy of each prior technology is taken up.
The multiplication of enlistment and synecdochic relationship between
imaging and photography also serves to invest greater power and authority in each subsequent technology.

Finally, in much the same way as subjective patient report is authorized
via neuroimaging detour, the recognition of the latest neuroimager as detour eligible is predicated on a prior CBD between imaging technologies.
The density of articulations that surround neuroimagers invest them with
the requisite authority to serve as sites of detour. The synecdochic relationship between medical imagers and cameras is a part of this. It reinforces the notion of medical imagers as objects that do representational
work. When the relationship between the vehicle and tenor was merely
metaphorical, medical imaging lacked much of the power it holds today.
Nowhere is this more apparent than in the case of the ontologization of
FMS, which I will address in the next chapter. As alluded to above, FMS

has long suffered from a state of illegitimacy. Despite the prevalence of clinical and patient report practices that stage an ontology of FMS, the mainstream medical establishment historically refused to grant the disorder metaphysical recognition. These (typically) women were seen as merely "crazy," as the passage interviewing Dr. Yunus attests above.

This particular CBD will be explored in great detail in the next chapter alongside my investigation of rarefactive calibration in the case of the sinus headache. However, before I do so, I must take one last short detour to address my ethical aporia regarding the CBD through neuroimaging to authorize subjective patient report. I am immediately struck by the presumptive need for authorization as an epiphenomenon of the two-world problem. Even among biopsychosocial advocates, the two-world of modernist biomedicine cannot be fully escaped. In the face of the manifest success of CBD through neuroimaging, ethical concerns persist. It is arguably a good thing that CBD through neuroimaging authorizes patient subjective report in cases of previously illegitimate diseases. Indeed, there is a long history of patients not receiving proper care for migraines and FMS. The ontologization of these diseases through CBD offers a great help in this regard. While fibromyalgics and migraineurs[1] manifestly benefit from CBD through neuroimaging, it is still an act of epistemic violence. Patient subjective report is still not trusted, and these patients still are not authorized to speak and be heard. Fibromyalgics and migraineurs are silenced once again as they are spoken for. Indeed, I am struck by the resonance between my account of neuroimaging technologies and Spivak's (1999) investigation of British colonists saving Indian women from ritual suicide. Spivak's locution involving "white men saving brown women from brown men" is uncomfortably paralleled in my narrative of white-coated men saving pained women from other white-coated men. As the neurosciences extend their domain into more and more areas of inquiry, purporting to explain the unexplained and represent the unrepresented, I'm not the first to think about the possible need for a postcolonial study of the neurosciences. Indeed, Bunge (2010) dubs the phenomenon "neuroimperialism." While I will return to this periodically in the chapters that follow, I cannot fully address it within the scope of this book. Nevertheless, I am compelled to raise the subject where I can, lest it be forgotten entirely.

CHAPTER FIVE

Rarefactive and Constitutive Calibration

The myth of "sinus" headache is perpetuated by the mass marketing of over-the-counter headache medications targeted at the large number of headache sufferers. —Michigan Headache Clinic, 2009

The concept of fibromyalgia has fallen into disrepute because it failed to overcome the essentialist fallacy that was the downfall of its predecessors, muscular rheumatism, neurasthenia, and fibrositis. — Quinter and Cohen, "Fibromyalgia Falls Foul of Fallacy"

Chances are if you owned a television in the last decade, you have seen a commercial for sinus headache medicine. Whether the product advertised was manufactured by Sudafed, Benadryl, or Excedrin, you were likely presented with a juxtaposition of pained people clutching their foreheads and fancy computerized animations showing yellow or red glowing pain areas relieved by flying blue or pink dots. This is, of course, a very familiar script in pharmaceutical advertising, especially for over-the-counter (OTC) analgesics. As a result of these advertisements, the sinus headache is a familiar illness in much of the English-speaking world. So it might be somewhat surprising to learn that the Michigan Headache Clinic decries the sinus headache as a myth. Fibromyalgia syndrome is obviously much less well known than the sinus headache. Nevertheless, in late June 2007, something very important happened for millions of chronic pain patients. The FDA approved Lyrica, a prescription drug originally developed as an anticonvulsant, for the treatment of FMS. In the world of contemporary biomedicine—an environment saturated by new drugs and regular FDA approvals—this may not seem like news. However, this particular FDA approval was especially interesting given the fact that until recently, as the second epigraph above indicates, much of the medical community did not even consider FMS a real disease. As such, the Lyrica approval functioned not only as a policy statement but also as an ontological pronouncement—that is, it codified the reality of FMS.

Taken together, the cases of the sinus headache and FMS provide an ideal opportunity to explore ontological change via calibration. In each of these cases, we find concerted disciplinary, political, and regulatory efforts to change the metaphysical status of a given disease. In the first case, the commonly accepted and arguably real sinus headache is declared a myth (no longer real). In the second case, a disease largely considered to be at best a psychiatric condition or at worst malingering is ushered into reality by the combined efforts of patient advocacy groups, rheumatologists, neurologists, and FDA regulators. A comparative examination of these two cases offers us the opportunity to explore two additional, but closely related, modes of calibration: rarefactive and constitutive, the terms I use to describe how the broader biomedical community works to bring diseases into or remove them from being. These are acts of calibration in that they coordinate diverse practical regimes of engagement and their emergent ontologies. In the case of the sinus headache, the practices of clinical otolaryngology and OTC self-medication stage an ontology where the sinus headache is a key player. In contrast, the scientific research practices of EBM and the clinical practices of neurology stage a closely related ontology with migraines at the center. Thus, the practices of otolaryngology, OTC self-medication, empirical-discursive medical science, and neurology must be calibrated to one another; when the conflict is irreconcilable, *rarefaction* results. The disease in question is removed from the ontology. Similarly, the clinical practices of rheumatology stage an ontology that includes FMS. However, the empirical-discursive practices of medical science, with their focus on variable isolation and control, stage an ontology of FMS as either nonexistent or mental illness. In the search for legitimacy, fibromyalgics and rheumatologists must calibrate their practices to the empirical-discursive in order to *constitute* a shared ontology.

While I remain committed to Mol's notion of multiple ontologies emergent in practice, I think cases such as these demonstrate the reciprocal interactions possible among local sites of practice, empirical-discursive ontologies, and regulatory structures. After all, medical practice does not occur in a vacuum. Doctors and patients cannot simply do whatever they please, and as such there are limits on the ontologies that can be staged. Clinical practice happens in highly regulated locales that function at the intersections among multiple disciplines and federal regulations. It is essential, therefore, to interrogate these two cases (FMS and the sinus head-ache) alongside each other, lest my analysis slide too easily into the hege-monic fallacy, the easy deployment of all-powerful actors in postmodern inquiry. Health practices are subject to limits, as the case of the sinus headache demonstrates. However, those limits are not totalizing. The case of FMS points to opportunities for agency and ontological change that the hegemonic fallacy would deny. The twin cases provide a necessary check on each other, neither allowing us to take one as representative and in so doing replicate either the hegemonic fallacy or Romantic, voluntarist no-tions of agency.

Thus, this chapter will proceed first by outlining its primary theoreti-cal contribution, the notion of "ontological rarefaction" and its two va-rieties, rarefactive calibration and constitutive calibration. In so doing, I will identify three primary principles of rarefaction (Foucault's term) that operationalize the empirical-discursive ontology. As it turns out, the very same principles of rarefaction are used both in the ontologization of FMS (constitutive calibration) and the de-ontologization of the sinus headache (rarefactive calibration). Finally, I will demonstrate how these principles of rarefaction are employed by "institutions of rarefaction" to police bio-medical ontologies.

Ontological Rarefaction

To begin, I turn first to Foucault's "Discourse on Language," in which he outlines several mechanisms for the regulation of discourse, terming them the "principles of rarefaction." As Foucault notes, "The produc-tion of discourse is at once controlled, selected, organised, and redis-tributed according to a certain number of procedures, whose role is to avert its powers and its dangers, to cope with change events, to evade its ponderous, awesome materiality" (1972, p. 216). These procedures are the principles of rarefaction, the mechanisms of control, selection, and organization. While both Foucault's language and my gloss of it highlight the restrictive action of principles of rarefaction, it is important to recog-nize their enabling function as well. Principles of rarefaction are those rules that govern discourse within certain systems. Certainly, they con-stitute a mechanism of control for aberrant discourse. However, at the same time as they inhibit heresy, they provide a legitimized forum for discourse that follows the rules.[1] Foucault's explanation of this facet of rarefaction is probably most clear in his discussion of speaking subjects (pp. 224–225). In this section of the "Discourse," he explains how within each system of discourse certain parties are recognized—granted permission to speak—while others are not.[2] Foucault describes the rarefaction of speaking subjects as a matter of qualification, and as such it could not be more appropriate for studies of medical discourse. The ability to contribute to (or speak in) medical discourse is controlled by a system of degrees, certifications, and fellowships. The quintuple-board-certified physician is automatically granted the right to pronounce on medical issues whereas marginalized speakers (chiropractors, midwifes, spiritual healers) are typically confined to other forums. In this sense, principles of rarefaction function as double-edged swords or flip sides of the same coin. Whichever your metaphor of choice, they simultaneously control some sources of discourse while enabling others.

In the "Discourse on Language," Foucault focuses primarily on seven principles of rarefaction—three external[3] to a given discourse and four internal. Certainly, madness, the will-to-truth, the author, disciplines, and the rarefaction of speaking subjects each have undergone significant scrutiny in rhetorical and cultural studies. However, these are not the principles that concern this chapter. As Foucault continues to explore principles of rarefaction, he alludes to unique principles that exist within each individual discursive system. Discussing disciplines, he writes, "Within its own limits every discipline recognizes true and false propositions. . . . In short, a proposition must fulfill some onerous and complex conditions before it can be admitted within a discipline; before it can be pronounced true or false it must be . . . 'within the true'"[4] (1972, pp. 223–224). Foucault's mandate that each proposition within a discourse must fulfill certain "onerous and complex conditions" applies readily to statements concerning the ontology and metaphysics of diseases. It is precisely these "onerous and complex conditions" that are the primary focus of this chapter and the engines of constitutive and rarefactive calibration. But first it is essential to note that principles of rarefaction do not spring into being from nowhere, especially in areas like medicine. Indeed, as Bourdieu (1988) argues in *Homo Academicus*, the more dangerous and powerful an area of inquiry, the more tightly regulated it must be:

> The faculty of law and the faculty of medicine, which, being able to provide the government with "the strongest and most durable influence on the people," are the most directly controlled by the government, the least autonomous from it

at the same time as the most directly entrusted with creating and controlling customary practice. (p. 62)

Here Bourdieu argues that medicine, extremely powerful and potentially dangerous, is not only regulated by its own disciplinary structures; it requires strenuous, strict regulation at the hands of the government. Certainly, this observation is borne out in contemporary America with organizations like the FDA and DEA wielding considerable oversight over medical discourse. Indeed, the FDA, charged with the regulation of pharmaceutical labeling—the regulation of a discourse—constitutes a prime example of an institution of rarefaction. Indeed, the federal government through the U.S. Food and Drug Act specifically charges the FDA with rarefactive duties, which will be investigated in greater detail in the next chapter.

Bourdieu's insight points to another important moment in Foucault's "Discourse" that is often ignored, but is critical for my analysis of constitutive and rarefactive calibration. Principles of rarefaction are implemented through the auspices of "institutions of rarefaction"—my term for the organizational or administrative locus of power from which principles of rarefaction derive. As Foucault explains, "The will-to-truth, like the other systems of exclusion, relies on institutional support: it is both reinforced and accompanied by whole strata of practices such as pedagogy—naturally—the book-system, publishing, libraries, such as the learned societies in the past, and laboratories today" (p. 219). Similarly, institutions of rarefaction such as the FDA, the DEA, journal editors, and professional medical organizations each deploy their own principles of rarefaction, and through them contribute substantively to the rarefaction of discourse.

In keeping with one of the primary goals of this book—the unification of rhetorical and new material approaches—I aim to avoid sole reliance on (new) material constructs such as principles of rarefaction. Rhetoricians, too, have well-established methodological resources that can contribute to this inquiry, a construct that explains the availability of common discursive resources that may be available to both constitutive and rarefactive calibration. Here I refer to the special topoi. Indeed, when one thinks back to Foucault's description of the differences between general principles of rarefaction—authority, disciplines, criticism—and those of the discipline-specific variety, the parallels between "The Discourse on Language" and Aristotle's *On Rhetoric* are striking:

But there are also those special *topoi* which are based on such propositions as apply only to particular groups or classes of things. Thus there are propositions about natural science on which it is impossible to base any enthymeme or syllogisms about ethics, and other propositions about ethics on which nothing can be based about natural science. The same principle applies throughout. The general *topoi* have no special subject-matter, and therefore will not increase our understanding of any particular class of things. (Aristotle, 1358b)

Ultimately, here, I am suggesting that one can regard principles of rarefaction as a special type of topos. Authority, disciplines, and criticism can be understood as common topoi that are available for use argumentatively within any discourse. Special topoi like specific etiology, diagnostic validity, and objective visualization may only be applicable to specific discourses such as those pertaining to disease.

However, merely identifying principles of rarefaction as topoi does not provide an exhaustive rhetorical account of the role of such principles in calibration. Principles of rarefaction must be a special type of topos in that not all topoi are capable of generating such persuasive and ontological force. Subsequently, I argue that principles of rarefaction should be understood as *warranting* topoi. Indeed, Toulmin's (2003) description of argumentative warrants is replete with the language of authority:

> Supposing we encounter this fresh challenge, we must bring forward not further data . . . but propositions of a rather different kind: rules, principles, inference-licenses or what you will, instead of additional items of information. Our task is no longer to strengthen the ground on which our argument is constructed, but is rather to show that, taking these data as a starting point, the step to the original claim or conclusion is an appropriate and legitimate one. . . . Propositions of this kind I shall call *warrants* (W), to distinguish them from both conclusions and data. (These "warrants," it will be observed correspond to the practical standards or canons of argument.) (Toulmin, 2003, p. 91)

Much like Aristotle's topoi, warrants are available resources that can be deployed in a variety of different argumentative contexts. However, their function as "rules, principles, inference-licenses" imbues them with an authorizing function within a given argument. Furthermore, Toulmin's metaphor—the warrant—makes the concept all the more applicable to principles of rarefaction. Warrants are documents of authority—authority derived from the judiciary and exercised by law enforcement. Similarly, as I argued above, principles of rarefaction are mechanisms of calibration (both constitutive and rarefactive) derived from disciplines (institutions of rarefaction) and exercised by peer reviewers. They are material-semiotic apparatuses that provide arguments (whether regulatory or agentive) with authorizing force.

Finally, there is one additional key parallel among principles of rarefaction, warrants, and the deployment of certain special topoi—their typical obfuscation. Speaking of the will-to-truth, Foucault (1972) suggests that focus on true facts engendered by the will-to-truth cannot help but to "mask" that will (p. 219). Furthermore, he argues that "we are unaware of the prodigious machinery of the will-to-truth" (p. 220). Generally speaking, principles of rarefaction are self-effacing. They are contrast background features exercising considerable control over discourse. Certainly the taboo against naming the will-to-truth, which Foucault references, is the prime example. As he argues, traditionally an identification of the will-to-truth would result in an exercise of the will-to-truth, and the identifier would be identified as mad or irrational. (Now the will-to-truth is the bedrock principle of modern empirical/scientific practices, and as such the taboo against its identification is perhaps stronger than other principles of rarefaction.) Indeed, principles of rarefaction are generally tacit unless they must be used explicitly in order to rarefy—to exorcise the aberrant discourse. This model of use is perfectly in keeping with Toulmin's description of warrants. Specifically, his theory uses a jurisprudential analogy to argue the case:

> The warrant is, in this sense, incidental and explanatory, its task being simply to register explicitly the legitimacy of the step involved to refer it back to the larger class of steps whose legitimacy is being presupposed. This is one of the reasons for distinguishing between data and warrants: data are appealed to explicitly, warrants implicitly. . . . This distinction, between data and warrants, is similar to the distinction drawn in law-courts between questions of fact and questions of law. (Toulmin, 2003, p. 1418)

This assumed or tacit nature of principles of rarefaction, warrants, and special topoi is part of what grants them such persuasive force. As a common point of reference within a discourse, they authorize claims—typically without interrogation. In Aristotelian logic, principles of rarefaction are the foundation of enthymematic argument. In Toulmin's schema, they are the (often) uninvoked warrant that legitimizes the use of the data to support the claim.[5] In combining principles of rarefaction with this notion of warranting topoi, I can better explain the power and authority of principles of rarefaction (their origin in institutions of rarefaction) and the rhetorical mechanism through which their use can be understood (warranting, enthymematic) as part of the practices of constitutive and rarefactive calibration. And this is precisely what I will do in the following sections as I explore how powerful principles of rarefaction at work in the practices of EBM serve to warrant the calibrating efforts of those seeking to either rarefy sinus headaches or constitute FMS.

Principles of Rarefaction

All told, the collected results from my investigations of FMS and the sinus headache reveal at least four principles of rarefaction/warranting topoi (PR/WT) at work that pertain specifically to ontological calibration of diseases. The cases suggest that in order to make a positive assertion concerning the ontological status of a disease (to claim that a disease *is*), one must have some combination of the following established under the scrutiny of various institutions of rarefaction:

1. An accepted specific etiology (biomechanistic cause)
2. Codified and statistically valid diagnostic criteria
3. Objective visual evidence
4. An FDA-approved treatment

These PR/WT suggest that the practical regimes of engagement that stage a given disease occur at the intersection of multiple different disciplines and institutions. For example, the establishment of a specific etiology typically occurs within the disciplinary boundaries of pathology, while statistical validation for diagnostics occurs within diagnostics journals. Furthermore, ontological rarefaction also occurs within nondisciplinary institutions such as the FDA. Subsequently, an interrogation of the constitutive and rarefactive disease calibration requires conceptualizing of such activities as an intersection or amalgamation of multiple institutions of rarefaction.

The long-standing material-semiotic investments in the practices of pathological inquiry provide the discipline of pathology (through the agency of its journals and professional boards) the power to calibrate disease ontologies. This power is exercised through recourse to PR/WT. Similarly, a diagnostician can cast doubt on the legitimacy of a disease by warranting his or her claims with the principle/topos of diagnostic validity. In short, if a diagnostic inventory has not been statistically validated, it will be cast out. In cases of doubt, a clinician or a researcher might CBD through radiology as described in the last chapter. And finally, an FDA indication for a specific drug to be used for a specific disease is an act of ontological calibration that links the empirical-discursive to the clinical regimes of practical engagement that stage that disease.

Ultimately, the discourses of FMS and the sinus headache suggest that specific etiology is the primary mechanism of ontological rarefaction of disease. And this, of course, makes sense given that pathology is literally the study of diseases. However, in the absence of authorized pathological data, researchers, clinicians, and/or pharmaceutical corporations lay claim to principles of rarefaction from diagnostics, radiology, and regulatory agencies in order to warrant their arguments. In the sections that follow, I will outline each of the first three identified principles of rarefaction, starting with specific etiology. Because the discussions of diagnostic validity and objective visualization overlap considerably with the sections on the semiotic pain ontology and CBD via neuroimaging in chapters 1 and 4, respectively, my treatment of them here will be brief. After outlining specific etiology and detail and clarifying my discussion of diagnostic validity and objective visualization, I will document the use of each of these PR/WT in the calibrating activities surrounding FMS and the sinus headache.

Specific Etiology and Pathogenesis

As the discipline primarily charged with the study and classification of disease, pathology—through the agency of its institutions of rarefaction (journal editors, professional organizations)—exerts considerable force over its ontology. Embodying Foucault's dictum that "for a discipline to exist, there must be the possibility of formulating—and doing so *ad infinitum*—fresh propositions" (p. 223), pathology conceives of itself very broadly. Textbooks of pathology often define themselves through recourse to etymology. For example, *Pathology for the Health Professions* (2006—a textbook designed for nonphysician health professionals) begins as follows:

> In this book you will read about pathology—the basic medical science concerned with diseases. The term *pathology* is derived from two Greek words: *pathos*, meaning disease, and *logos*, meaning science. Thus, pathology is the science that studies diseases. (Damjanov, 2006, p. xiii)

However, the polyphony of ancient Greek means that pathology means different things to different English-speaking people. In contrast, a prominent physician-oriented text defines pathology as follows:

> Pathology is literally the study (*logos*) of suffering (*pathos*). More specifically, it is a bridging discipline involving both basic science and clinical practice and is devoted to the study of the structural and functional changes in cells, tissues, and organs that underlie disease. By the use of molecular, microbiologic, immunologic, and morphologic techniques, pathology attempts to explain the whys and wherefores of the signs and symptoms manifested by patients while providing a sound foundation for rational clinical care and therapy. (Kumar, Abbas & Fausto, 2005, p. 4)

Certainly each of these definitions carves out a large space for pathological discourse. However, just because a discipline allows for an infinite number of statements does not mean that those statements can be of infinite kind. As previously acknowledged, institutions of rarefaction employ principles of rarefaction in order to legitimize some discourse and restrict others. Although pathology's institutions marshal a variety of PR/WT, the doctrines of specific etiology and pathogenesis are primary.

In surveying about a dozen pathology textbooks,[6] I found that all of them followed the basic definition (study of disease) by articulating these two subdisciplinary spheres. One representative example reads as follows:

> The primary goal of this book is to teach you the basic concepts underlying various pathologic processes. You will study the *pathogenesis* of diseases, learn their mechanisms, and understand how they develop. You will learn the *etiology* of pathologic changes and understand the causes of many diseases. (Damjanov, 2006, p. xiii)

Pathogenesis and etiology are the cornerstones of so-called modern pathology, which owes its origin to late nineteenth-century German physician Rudolf Virchow. Virchow is largely credited with the establishment of contemporary (often called "microscopic") pathology. His initial work involved the identification of the syphilis bacterium (1848). Since modern pathology was inaugurated through microscopic practices that stage an ontology of the study of a disease with a metaphysics of isolable pathogen, the doctrine of specific etiology's focus on monocausality was all but assured. Furthermore, as a product of its empirical-discursive ontology and biomechanical metaphysics, modern pathology's focus on causality and mechanistic explanation is, no doubt, part of the reason that pathology can exert so much control over disease discourse. The doctrines of specific etiology and pathogenesis coordinate very effectively with the mechanistic metaphysics that ground modernist scientific inquiry.

Of course, the doctrine of specific etiology and its focus on monocausality has been broadly criticized by medical humanists and critical scholars of health (Elliott, 2003; Whitbeck, 1981; Engelhardt, 1976). Furthermore, those invested in a holistic approach, like the biopsychosocial pain scientists and clinicians discussed in previous chapters, have argued that disease is invariably multicausal, and the focus of isolable single causes is inappropriate. Even the explicitly mechanistic textbooks acknowledge this concern. The 2005 edition of a prominent medical school pathology textbook notes:

> The concept, however, of one etiologic agent for one disease—developed from the study of infections or single-gene disorders—is no longer sufficient. Genetic factors are clearly involved in some of the common environmentally induced maladies, such as atherosclerosis and cancer, and the environment may also have profound influences on certain genetic diseases. (Kumar, Abbas & Fausto, 2005, p. 4)

Of course, this passage is immediately followed by a move to simply ignore this very problem: "Knowledge or discovery of *the primary cause* remains the backbone on which diagnosis can be made, a disease understood, or a treatment developed" (p. 4, emphasis added). And the remainder of the textbook pretty much focuses on "*the* etiologic agent" for each disease.

While this criticism is of great concern for pain practitioners and medical ethicists, it is also this very issue that gives pathology so much legitimizing force in calibrating disease. In ontologies staged by traditional scientific inquiry, mechanistic causality and isolable variables are the norm. Complex systems modeling methodologies that stage ontologies of multicausality are relatively new and are only taking hold in those disciplines that require them to produce results (for example, predictive climate modeling, ecology, agronomy). Medicine, in contrast, is often attributed with tremendous popular success because of the way it isolates disease agents and cures them.

As such, without a clearly identified and disciplinarily legitimized pathogenesis and etiology, it is very difficult to make authoritative claims concerning a disease. As Aho (2008) notes in his exploration of contemporary psychiatric diagnostics:

> Bio-psychiatry interprets mental disorders from the same objectifying and mechanistic perspective that modern science inherited from the philosophies of Descartes and his empiricist successors. This perspective already makes pre-judgments about what is valuable. [This perspective] adopts a mechanistic picture of the world as an aggregate of quantifiable material objects in causal interaction. (p. 249)

This mechanistic view into which biopsychiatry is articulated also exerts its sway over medical practices, scientific and clinical. As medicine was subsumed by scientific practices such as microscopy, the emergent mechanistic metaphysics of the two-world problem began to take hold. In this metaphysics, the ultimate mark of understanding is mechanistic description—or in medicine pathogenesis (or pathophysiology) and etiology. The result of all this is that the requirement of an articulable pathogenesis and etiology is a very powerful PR/WT. Being able to demonstrate convincingly the pathogenesis and etiology of a disease firmly places that disease in the realm of truth and allows one to make authoritative ontological claims about it.

Diagnostic Criteria and Predictive Validity

In contemporary medicine, the practices of diagnostics and pathology have nearly collapsed into one. If medical science can locate an empirically isolable component of a specific etiology (for example, a chemical marker in the blood or a medical image), then the clinician can locate that marker in a patient, and a diagnostic pronouncement can be made. From antiquity to the present, diagnosis has been understood as the practice of reading signs and symptoms in order to arrive at a label for a patient's affliction. However, in cases when the disease in question has been recently identified or resists the logic of the specific etiology (that is, is multicausal or based on subjective patient report), then clinicians are forced to rely on a different set of practices for identifying and classifying illness. Chapter 1 of this book offers a more complete exploration of the practices of diagnosis and pain's semiotic ontology. As I explained, contemporary diagnosis is grounded in statistical practices underscored by the discourses of EBM. It is the statistical ground from which these diagnoses are derived that gives them so much rarefactive force in ontological calibration. Relevant and predictive diagnostic signs and symptoms are carefully and painstakingly researched in order to arrive at a robust diagnostic inventory. Indeed, evaluating the reliability of diagnostic tests is a lively research agenda, as would be expected given the newfound reliance on probability tables. As noted in *Designing Clinical Research* (2013):

> For a test to be useful it must pass muster on a series of increasingly difficult questions that address its *reproducibility, accuracy, feasibility,* and *effects on clinical decisions* and *outcomes.* Favorable outcomes to each of these questions are necessary but insufficient criteria for a test to be worth doing. For example, if a test does not give consistent results when performed by different people or in different places, it can hardly be useful. If the test seldom supplies new information and hence seldom affects clinical decisions, it may not be worth doing. Even if it affects decisions, if these decisions do not improve the clinical outcome of patients who were tested, the tests still may not be useful. (Hulley et al., 2013, p. 183, emphasis in original)

The primary source of evidence for the "reproducibility, accuracy," and "feasibility" of (especially pain-related and psychological) diagnostic inventories are diagnostic validity studies. A form of calibration in their own right, diagnostic validity studies articulate subjective patient report on disciplining inventories to pathological findings. Of course, this is a form of buttressing, as I suggested in chapter 3. And as I alluded to in the last chapter and will further describe below, frequently in cases like FMS the PR/WT of objective visualization is employed to further legitimize the diagnosis as a result of subjective patient report.

Objective Visualization

The role of visualization and visualization technologies in contemporary biomedical practices is so extensive and nuanced that it has fostered a rich body of critical literature in fields ranging from STS to medical anthropology. Indeed, these issues are addressed in great detail in the previous chapter. The authority invested in neuroimaging technologies through CBD offers one account of the power they hold in contemporary efforts of ontological calibration. In this chapter, I continue this discussion by arguing that visualization technology is able to exert its authority in ontological rarefaction precisely because the series of detouring calibrations that articulate novel imaging technologies extends all the way back to the medical gaze and the ocular centrism that underlies all of Western scientific practices. As such, the ability to "see" something *via* medical imaging functions as a PR/WT. As Haraway (1997) explains, visualization technologies are routinely responsible for bringing scientific objects into the true:

> Both the whole earth and the fetus owe their existence as public objects to visualizing technologies. . . . The system of ideological oppositions between signifiers of touch and vision remains stubbornly essential to political and scientific debate in modern Western culture. (p. 174)

Employing the speculum as synecdoche, Haraway argues that visualization technologies that allow the scientific gaze to penetrate previously hidden spaces are often responsible for the acceptance of the reality of the described objects that exist in those hidden spaces. Medical imaging is a prime exemplar of a high-technology speculum, and Haraway's virtual speculum synecdoche is so obviously apropos for imaging technologies that the correspondence between the vehicle and the tenor hardly bears mentioning. It is the strong historical links among visualization technologies, ocular centrism, and the metaphysics of presence that make objective visualization such an important PR/WT in the discourses of constitutive and rarefactive calibration.

Sinus Headache Rarefaction

I first witnessed rarefactive calibration in regard to the sinus headache while attending a 2007 meeting of the MPG. The speaker—the aforementioned quintuple-board-certified physician with expertise in internal medicine, anesthesiology, pain medicine, and headaches—declared that the sinus headache was a myth, that it was invented and promulgated by pharmaceutical advertising (MPG Journal Club, February 2007). As someone who has seen plenty of sinus headache advertisements and even been told once or twice by my GP that I had a sinus headache, I was a bit skeptical. However, subsequent research has done little but validate the MPG speaker's argument. Dr. Dana Winegarner of what was then known as the MidAmerican Neuroscience Institute refers to sinus headaches as "a popular myth" (MidAmerican Neuroscience Institute, n.d.). An article in the journal *Headache*, a publication of the American Headache Society, refers to the sinus headache as "the most frequent erroneous diagnosis given to patients with migraine" (Eross, Dodick & Eross, 2007, p. 214). Multiple sources suggest the expansion in sinus headache medicine advertising has come along with a concomitant increase in sinus headache diagnoses from patients and clinicians alike. As one article from *WebMD* puts it, "Sinus headache: we are the only country in the world that sees a significant health problem in this. . . . I think part of this is Madison Avenue convincing us of something that is more accurately part of a migraine" (DeNoon, 2003). This sentiment was echoed by the February 2007 MPG speaker who presented epidemiological data that showed the highest prevalence of sinus headache to be in the United States, Germany, and Sweden—the three countries in which sinus headache medicine has the largest advertising budget. In each of these cases, health-care providers place the blame largely on the marketing and advertising arms of the pharmaceutical corporations. In suggesting that the sinus headache is not a disease, authors often invoke a principle of rarefaction in their argument. For example, the following excerpt highlights two of the major principles in one sentence:

> Sinus headache is the most frequent erroneous diagnosis given to patients with migraine. This diagnostic confusion is based in part on the paucity of nosologic research to define the distinguishing clinical features of headache associated with rhino-sinus pathology, and the lack of operational diagnostic criteria. (Eross, Dodick & Eross, 2007, p. 214)

This objection to sinus headache focuses on (1) the lack of an acceptable pathological foundation (specific etiology) and (2) the lack of legitimized diagnostic criteria. Each of these are points of objection that warrant the authors' claims that the sinus headache is an illegitimately identified disease. Accordingly, we see specific etiology and valid diagnostic criteria functioning as PR/WT as part of the rarefactive calibration of the sinus headache.

Sinus Headache Pathology

Pathogenetic and etiological concerns are of primary importance in the debates surrounding the sinus headache. This is particularly so given the concern over "confusion" between sinus headache and migraines. Each side of the sinus headache debate warrants their claims with different pathophysiological and etiological arguments. The OTC pharmaceutical manufacturers' suggested etiology and pathogenesis is probably best represented by their graphical depictions of sinus suffering. These computer-graphics-driven advertisements depict increases in sinus congestion that result in pain and pressure around the eyes and nose. Despite the claim that the sinus headache is a relatively new invention of the pharmaceutical industry, it turns out the mechanisms behind the sinus headache have been theorized as early as 1891 (McBride, 1900).

Those who object to the existence of the sinus headache, or at least suggest that it is vastly overdiagnosed, also frequently rely on specific etiology and pathogenesis. In contrast to the pro–sinus headache group, these critics warrant their claims by citing the pathology of migraines. For example, Mehle and Schreiber (2005) ask in an article in *Otolaryngology*:

> Why are so many "sinus headache" patients misdiagnosed, either by their physicians or themselves? The answer to this question likely is related to the pathophysiology of migraine, and the nature of nasal pain. (p. 490)

Neurologists suggest that a brain structure known as the descending nucleus of five is built in such a way that when a patient has a migraine, it produces symptoms that resemble a sinus problem. As MPG speaker Dr. Heisenberg explained at a members meeting:

> If you look at the descending nucleus of five, the nucleus of pain is spread out over a space. It's not just a small group of cells. And unfortunately it is interweaved with this lower portion of the nucleus which are actually inputs from the back of the head for sensation and pain. Also very close by are nuclei that control [sinus- and congestion-related] symptoms. So it's easy to understand why we get so many of these look-alike syndromes in migraines. (February 2007)

According to Dr. Heisenberg, the neurological structures that control migraine headache are so intertwined with those that control sinus congestion that the former often causes the latter. In this case, sinus headaches are viewed as epiphenomena of migraines. Under the mechanistic rubric of pathology, this argument suggests that migraines cause the symptoms of sinus headaches. In offering an alternate specific etiology and pathogenesis, Dr. Heisenberg lays claim to the same PR/WT in order to reject the ontology of the sinus headache.

Sinus Headache Diagnosis

The problem of diagnosis is especially pertinent in the case of the sinus headache due to the argument about the confusion with migraines. Furthermore, even physicians who accept the legitimacy of the sinus headache cite the challenge in rendering the diagnosis. For example, in *Current Pain and Headache Reports*, Hauser and Levine identify the symptoms of sinus headache as "often vague, creating a challenge for the clinician in establishing an accurate diagnosis" (2008, p. 45). Diagnosing a sinus headache requires the comparison of patient symptoms with authorized diagnostic criteria, but the criteria are conflicting. The most broadly recognized is probably the criteria provided by the pharmaceutical industry. However, the most broadly authorized (by medico-scientific discourse) criteria are those provided by the International Headache Society (IHS). As the aforementioned *Current Pain and Headache Reports* article notes, the "IHS criteria are consensus-driven guidelines that categorize headaches into various subsets based on history and symptoms" (Hauser & Levine, 2008, p. 45). The IHS provides diagnosticians with five criteria for identifying a sinus headache:

> (1) purulent discharge of the nasal passages; (2) pathologic findings on x-ray examination, CT, magnetic resonance imaging (MRI) or transillumination; (3) simultaneous onset of headache and sinusitis; (4) headache location (in relationship to specific sinus structures); and (5) disappearance of headache after treatment of acute sinusitis. . . . The evidence for the importance of headache location in relationship to sinus disease is now considered doubtful, and the circular reasoning of the fifth criterion has been criticized. (Cady et al., 2005, p. 909)

The strictness of these criteria is often used as the justification for excluding the majority of patients from the sinus headache diagnosis and offering migraine as an alternative. These criteria position sinus headache as secondary to acute sinusitis, a viral or bacteriological condition. The alternative diagnostic criteria make the sinus headache much easier to diagnose, as they describe it as almost any head or facial pain resulting from sinus pressure.

One of the primary advocates of these criteria is the National Headache Foundation, an organization funded by an unrestricted educational grant from Eli Lilly. It should be acknowledged that these criteria, like the commercial advertisements, are geared more toward self-diagnosis than physician diagnosis, though they are used by quite a number of clinicians:

> Sinuses are filled with air, and their secretions must be able to drain freely into the nose. If your headache is truly caused by a sinus blockage, such as an infection, you will probably have a fever. (National Headache Foundation, 2008)

In the wake of diagnostic difficulties, clinicians often turn to diagnostic inventories that operate as part of the diagnostic-statistical ontology, and the sinus headache is no exception. Of course, each diagnostic approach to these headaches comes with a different specified inventory. If clinicians think of the sinus headache as a legitimate otolaryngologic disorder, then that will lead them to use an inventory such as the sinal-nasal outcomes test (SNOT-20, seriously) (Mehle & Schreiber, 2005, p. 490). However, if clinicians believe it to be primarily a migraine disorder, then there are appropriate migraine alternatives. This following excerpt reprinted from chapter 3 highlights the difficulty involved in selecting the appropriate diagnostic inventory, even for one illness (in this case migraine):

> So one of the things that is also an item of debate is which questionnaire to use. Oh gosh, does this sound familiar to psychologists? Which questionnaire should you use? There's actually an extraordinarily simple questionnaire called the HIT-6, and we haven't brought that to the group for a while, but that was promulgated by Glaxo. But nonetheless, it covers all areas of function. MIDAS actually only covers a few . . . it doesn't really cover energy. It doesn't ask you cognition questions. You, as a clinician, actually have to imply that in your questioning. It's kind of good to talk to the patient, besides just having them fill out a form. And emotional distress isn't covered. The most commonly used study methodology when determining severity of migraine disability is actually [MIDAS], in almost all the studies that are published now, even though there are actually better questionnaires in terms of covering everything. So, we need to see some further developments along this line. (MPG Journal Club, February 2007)

In an era where the reliability and validity of a diagnosis exercises tremendous rarefactive force, the question as to which test[7] to use is essential. Different tests offer clinicians different statistical resources in order to determine a diagnosis. Certain tests are more likely to result in one diagnosis over another, and frequently many tests are required. For example, the SNOT-20 will determine how likely it is that a given patient has a sinus headache. If the results are not significant, then the clinician may resort to the MIDAS or the HIT-6 in an effort to provide a different diagnosis.

Visualizing Sinus Headaches

While pathology and diagnostics exert considerable rarefaction control over disease ontology, objective visualization can function as a principle of last resort. While a clinician may not be able to identify the patho-physiology, and may not yet have identified statistically valid diagnostic criteria, if evidence for the disease can be "seen," then it is much harder to object to its reality. Visualization's foundation in ocular centrism certainly helps to provide those who employ it a certain legitimacy that they other-wise might not have. Subsequently, the principle of objective visualization is invoked in the sinus headache literature. Proponents of the sinus head-ache often point to radiographic findings to indicate the presence of an actual ailment, even in the absence of symptomology commensurate with the IHS criteria. Visualization technologies that subsume diagnostics un-der the logic of the gaze are common recourse for sinus ailment diagnos-tics. As the aforementioned *Current Pain and Headache* article describes:

> The nasal cavity is then carefully evaluated, often with an endoscope looking for pathology or anatomic abnormalities that may be the source of the symp-tomology. A CT scan of the sinuses is often obtained to better evaluate the anatomy and pathology. For patients with new-onset headaches and/or change in headache and/or facial pain character, an MRI of the head and sinuses is also obtained to look for sinister causes of the pain. (Hauser & Levine, 2008, p. 45)

In keeping with the pharmaceutically driven definition of the sinus head-ache (the one that includes many more patients), the National Headache Foundation downplays the IHS criteria (fever-inducing sinusitis) using the word "probably" and highlights the role of X-ray as unquestionable arbiter of diagnosis:

> Sinuses are filled with air, and their secretions must be able to drain freely into the nose. If your headache is truly caused by a sinus blockage, such as an infec-tion, you will probably have a fever. An x-ray will confirm a sinus blockage. (National Headache Foundation, 2008)

This recourse to visualization technologies is evident in more mainstream medical texts as well. An editorial titled "The Demise of the Sinus Headache Is Premature," published in the *Archives of Internal Medicine*, cites "the predictive value of headache for an abnormal CT finding in chronic sinusitis" (Chester, 2005, p. 954).

Similarly, a 2008 research study in *Headache*, the journal of the American Headache Society, uses radiological evidence to question the dichotomy between sinus headache and migraine:

> The majority of "sinus headache" patients satisfy the IHS criteria for migraine. Surprisingly, these patients often have radiographic sinus disease. This raises the possibility of selection bias in otolaryngology patients, inaccurate diagnosis, or radiographic sinus disease and migraine as comorbid conditions. (Mehle & Kremer, 2008, p. 67)

A more recent article in *Rhinology* argues that visualization should be contraindicated when the primary symptom is facial/sinus pain (Amir, Yeo & Ram, 2012). Indeed, the authors further present the results of a metastudy indicating that there is actually a poor correlation between facial pain and sinus pressure. The study notes that only 18 percent of patients with nasal pain had positive findings of sinus blockage and that of patents with sinus blockage, only 29 percent complained of pain.

In each of these cases, the work of institutions of rarefaction, through their PR/WT, can be seen. The disciplines of pathology, diagnostics, and radiology use the force of specific etiology, statistical validity, and objective visualization to rarefy the ontology of the sinus headache. For the most part, the tide seems to be turning against sinus headache. The etiological arguments suggesting that migraines are often mistaken as sinus headaches no longer bear the burden of proof. The diagnostic and radiological arguments largely support the pathological redefinition. Each disciplinary discourse has challenged the simple identification of headache and facial pain as an uncomplicated epiphenomenon of sinus congestion. The success of such rarefactive efforts is manifest in a variety of spheres. Some articles use scare quotes to denote the tenuousness of the "sinus headache" (Mehle & Kramer, 2008). Others now offer quite unwieldy constructions like "migraine presenting as sinus-headache" (Ishkanian, Blumenthal, Webster, Richardson & Ames, 2007). Perhaps the clearest evidence for the success of the rarefactive campaign comes from the occasional rebranding of some OTC sinus headache medicines as "sinus and pain" or "pressure and pain."

In sum, the case of the sinus headache provides an excellent illustration of rarefactive calibration in action. The medical community has succeeded, largely, in curtailing the efforts of the pharmaceutical community to market a drug for a disease that is not properly staged by the practices of medicine research. Indeed, as I have argued elsewhere (Graham, 2011), this is a positive finding in the face of overwhelming concerns that big pharmaceuticals are running roughshod over the U.S. regulatory process, an issue I will return to in chapter 6. However, first I must address constitutive calibration in the discourse of FMS. In so doing, I will demonstrate how FMS was successfully integrated into both the medical and the regulatory community, and further that that integration relied on the very same institutions and PR / WT that were used to block the sinus headache.

Constituting Fibromyalgia

Although some trace the issue back as far as Galen (circa 150 CE), the ontology of FMS has been a matter of intense debate for at least the past thirty years. As recently as the late 1990s, it was not uncommon to find medical literature strongly questioning the validity of this disorder. Indeed, the opening epigraph to this chapter from the prominent British medical journal the *Lancet* is quite damning. While my focus here is primarily on FMS as an exemplar of constitutive calibration, it is essential to recognize—all too briefly—the significant patient ramifications regarding patient care that arise from contested diseases. The president of a national FMS research and advocacy organization, herself a fibromyalgic, summed it up well during a participant interview: "Living with a chronic illness is challenging. Living with a chronic illness that people don't believe in is overwhelming—at best" (Martinez, ethnographic interview). Indeed, Martinez even cited the existence of numerous cases of fibromyalgic suicide that resulted, at least in part, from the climate of disbelief.

However, when one looks to more recent popular press or professional medical journals, one thing seems clear: Fibromyalgia is enjoying an increasing reality. The online information fact sheet provided by the Mayo Clinic unquestioningly classifies fibromyalgia as "a chronic condition characterized by widespread pain in your muscles, ligaments and tendons, as well as fatigue and multiple tender points—places on your body where slight pressure causes pain." And while the ability to provide such a succinct definition is quite new, the growing acceptance of FMS is bluntly confirmed in the following excerpt from an MPG meeting devoted to the subject:

DR. HEISENBERG (CLINICAL NEUROLOGIST): Are you aware of anyone who doesn't believe in fibromyalgia anymore?

DR. FITZPATRICK (ACADEMIC NEUROPHYSIOLOGIST): Not really. Maybe a few nut jobs.

DR. HEISENBERG: At least everyone pretty much agrees the pain is *real* now?

DR. FITZPATRICK: Oh yeah. Absolutely. (Journal Club presentation, February 2008)

This growing acceptance and the 2007 FDA approval of the first FMS drug is a rather inarguable index of change. As such, an inquiry into FMS's on-tologization provides an excellent counter case to that of the sinus head-ache. As promised above, the following sections will demonstrate the twin nature of constitutive and rarefactive calibration by documenting how the ontologization of FMS was accomplished through recourse to the same PR/WT that served to delegitimize the sinus headache.

Diagnosing FMS

A 2000 article from the *Philadelphia Inquirer* explains clearly the once great difficulty in obtaining an FMS diagnosis: "There are no objective markers of fibromyalgia—nothing that X-rays, blood tests, muscle bi-opsies or MRIs can find. For many patients fibromyalgia goes together with two other hard-to-diagnose syndromes: chronic fatigue and irritable bowel" (McCullough, 2000, p. D01). The practical and therefore eviden-tiary anxiety created by a lack of clear diagnostic criteria once pervaded FMS discourse. Although in the following passages we will see patients and clinicians oscillating between indexical and statistical diagnostic on-tologies, the anxiety remains. The symptoms do not point. The validity tables do not clarify. As fibromyalgia patient Anne explained in an in-terview with the *Globe and Mail*, "It can be tough to diagnose. . . . It depends on which specialist you see, what your presenting symptoms are" ("Causes of fibromyalgia," 2002, p. H1). Similarly, nationally re-nowned fibromyalgia specialist Dr. Daniel Clauw reported in an interview with the *Washington Times*, "There are still a number of people who are skeptical. . . . It is part of a spectrum of illness that falls into a gray zone, with no evidence on lab tests" (Goff, 2002, p. D1).

Without the PR/WT of legitimized and validated diagnostic criteria, it is quite difficult for FMS to be recognized within the discourse of diagnos-tics and medical science more broadly. Responding to this great concern, the American College of Rheumatology (ACR) convened meetings in the late 1980s in an effort to establish new accepted and validated diagnostic

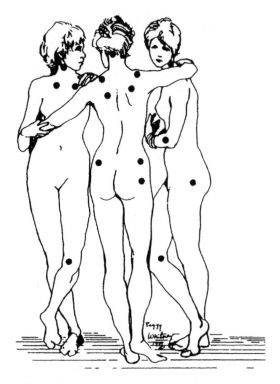

FIGURE 5.1. ACR fibromyalgia diagnostic criteria tender points. The broad bodily distribution of these tender points has provided FMS researchers with additional evidence of neurological dysregulation. Reprinted by permission from Wolfe et al. (1990).

criteria (see fig. 5.1) for FMS, to link FMS to the PR / WT of diagnostic medicine. The result was the now widely used (though not entirely accepted) tender-point criteria:

1. History of widespread pain.
   Definition. Pain is considered widespread when all of the following are present: pain in the left side of the body, pain in the right side of the body, pain above the waist, and pain below the waist. In addition, axial skeletal pain (cervical spine or anterior chest or thoracic spine or low back) must be present. In this definition, shoulder and buttock pain is considered as pain for each involved side. "Low back" pain is considered lower segment pain.
2. Pain in 11 of 18 tender point sites on digital palpation.
   Definition. Pain, on digital palpation, must be present in at least 11 of the following 18 sites: [sites listed]. (Wolfe et al., 1990)

Pursuant to this redefinition of FMS diagnostic criteria, any patient meeting the above criteria (both a history of widespread pain and pain at eleven of eighteen pre-identified tender points) can be classified as a fibromyalgic. Since 1990, these criteria "have been widely used, especially in clinical trials and epidemiological studies. These criteria have stimulated research on fibromyalgia worldwide, but are increasingly recognized to lack sensitivity for diagnosis in clinical settings" (Perrot, Dickenson & Bennett, 2008, p. 2).

Here we see the beginnings of constitutive calibration made possible by leveraging a PR/WT. The clinical practices of rheumatology are codified in the form of the tender-point criteria, which are then deployed in medical research under the empirical-discursive ontology. The practical effect of these new criteria in stimulating more research into FMS certainly paved the way for its acceptance.

Even with the broad adoption of the 1990 ACR FMS criteria, clinicians and researchers still suffered from the epistemological uncertainties that arose from the dearth of biomechanically legitimized FMS evidence. However, the 1990 ACR criteria did (unintentionally) provide a theoretical framework that legitimized a new place to look for that missing evidence. In the editorial "Fibromyalgia Is Not a Rheumatologic Disease Anymore," Griffing (2008) explains how the tender-point research that followed the adoption of the ACR criteria proved rather conclusively that "tender points have nothing to do with fibromyalgia" (p. 47). It does not necessarily take a medical expert to see the next logical development in FMS research. If FMS causes widespread bodily pain and is not caused at the pain locations, then FMS is likely a nervous system (spine or brain) problem. In fact, most literature now classifies FMS as a central nervous system (CNS) disorder, making it perhaps more the providence of neurologists than rheumatologists. (And thus we see another possible example of neuroimperialism.)

Visualizing FMS

With the reclassification of FMS as a CNS disorder, researchers renewed their etiological investigations—this time with the brain as primary focus. And of course, as discussed in the last chapter, contemporary biomedical studies of the brain regularly turn to ubiquitous and powerful neuroimaging technologies to "see" the phenomena under study. From the popular *Newsweek* to the scholarly *Rheumatology*, neuroimaging technologies have been hailed for filling the evidentiary gap inhibiting the study of FMS. The literature is filled with a litany of one-liners exclaiming the persuasive impact of neuroimaging data. Although the generic conventions of popular press accounts allow for more provocative stylistics—for example, "Thanks to brain-scan technology, this 'imaginary' ailment of 6 million people is proving to be very real" (Underwood, 2003, p. 53)—there is also a certain excitement and anticipation in academic accounts:

> These recent applications of functional neuroimaging have provided evidence for a centralized pain augmentation in FMS and identified brain regions that may be involved in this augmentation. Advances in design and new imaging technologies promise to further increase our understanding of the mechanisms that initiate and maintain this disorder and can lead to improved diagnosis and treatment. (Williams & Gracely, 2006, p. 231)

One can look also to the following excerpt from *Chemist and Druggist*. Not only is neuroimaging noted for providing the first clear-cut biomechanical evidence of FMS—imaging technologies have also taken center stage in convincing the medical community of the reality of FMS:

> Fibromyalgia is an enigma. No one disputes that patients experience considerable pain and distress, but the pain is diffuse, there is no obvious pathology in particularly tender areas. . . . Many clinicians traditionally regarded fibromyalgia as predominately psychosomatic, rather than neurological or physiological. However, advances over recent years might be on the verge of resolving these pathophysiological and therapeutic enigmas. For example, imaging studies reveal several differences in the brains of people with fibromyalgia compared to controls. ("Pharmacy Update," 2007, p. 17)

The long-standing debate over the ontology of FMS has created an environment of epistemological uncertainty among pain management and FMS clinicians. Even those clinicians who are convinced of the existence of FMS hedge their statements about it and point out some of the problems in the data. In my work with pain management clinicians, I frequently observed health-care providers stipulate FMS's existence while highlighting the lack of evidence.

The debate over the ontology of FMS led Dr. Heisenberg, in a presentation to the MPG in February 2008, to express doubts about the entire epistemology of neuroscience medicine:

> One of the things I want to talk about before [I begin] is the philosophical stance of this whole business of fibromyalgia. . . . I'm going to just cover a little

bit about the whole aspect of looking at the universe of medical ideas, and one of the problems that we have is that we always have this disappearing, reverberating situation with this homunculus. Do you all know what a homunculus is? It's a sensory system. [It describes, through systems-modeling, neurological functions.] The point is that there is a disappearing or always receding homunculus problem, philosophically. When you're trying to scoop up something and say that it's there, and all that you have is a bit of circular reasoning. . . . So if we try to describe a state, like chronic pain, we're going to assume it's a state of consciousness that must experience the pain. And of course the problem is we don't even know how to describe consciousness. I'm just mentioning the classic Pascal-Gödel conundrum for math: You can't describe any system unless you posit at least one thing outside of the system. You cannot complete it. You can't prove it, without one thing. As my old philosophy professor used to say, "Give me a Coke can; give me a bedpost; give me anything. If you absolutely guarantee me you're going to say that exists, I can prove the rest of the universe." You gotta start somewhere. So the consciousness epiphenomenon is just a part of this receding homunculus thing. Where you're always describing something else with another, but more complex, thing you can't actually name or doubt. (MPG Journal Club, February 2008)

In the preceding quotation, which tacitly recognizes the iterative and cyclical nature of CBD in neurology, Dr. Heisenberg expresses his concern that neuroscience modeling is built on an ever-receding set of homunculi. That is, every description of a neurological system is predicated on another system that has been essentially black boxed for the sake of the current model. Subsequently, when describing complex neurological systems such as pain processing, neuroscientists are faced with an inherent problem of infinitely receding homunculi, or in the more familiar parlance of philosophers, we have once again a situation where it is turtles/homunculi/black boxes all the way down. This is, of course, a very challenging proposition for medical practitioners whose work is often built on a foundation of "pretended omniscience" (Turner, 1990, p. 192). Nevertheless, this epistemological anxiety vis-à-vis FMS provides an ideal entrée for neuroimaging data. In essence, neuroimaging has provided the first "real" object that can function as the Archimedean data point to legitimize the entire discourse of FMS. Neuroimaging data is Dr. Heisenberg's Coke can or bedpost.

To date, neuroimaging research has provided quite a few insights into FMS and subsequently provided a foundation for further ontologizing the disorder. As one article in *Pain Practice* notes in regard to imaging technology, "Advances in technology have led to a better understanding of the pathophysiology of FMS, including the key role of disordered pain processing in its symptomology" (Perrot, Dickenson & Bennett, 2008, p. 10). Another article from *Arthritis Research and Therapy* offers several paragraphs enumerating the valuable FMS insights gained from PET, beginning as follows:

> These recent applications of functional neuroimaging have provided evidence for a centralized pain augmentation in FMS and identified brain regions that may be involved in this augmentation. Advances in design and new imaging technologies promise to further increase our understanding of the mechanisms that initiate and maintain this disorder and can lead to improved diagnosis and treatment. (Williams & Gracely, 2006, p. 231)

Returning to the language of rhetorical-ontological inquiry, ontologizing FMS can be described as a process of constitutive CBD. Laboratory diagnostic practices are incapable of staging an ontology of FMS that matches the ontology staged by subjective patient report. Subsequently, rheumatologists and patients use the ACR criteria to detour through the black box of neuroimaging, and in so doing calibrate the clinical ontology of FMS to the practices of EBM and objective visualization. The 1990 ACR criteria provided clinicians with a constellation of partially authorized statements that they could make about FMS, although these statements were still without ontological foundation. Neuroimaging, by virtue of its authorizing foundation in objective visualization, provided FMS researchers and clinicians with access to a legitimized object, and thus the object—by way of the neuroimaging—legitimized the discourse of FMS. However, the full realization of this constitutive CBD cannot be seen until the practices of clinical rheumatology, diagnostics, and objective visualization are calibrated to the practices of biomedical pathology.

FMS Pathology

In spite of the broad success and power of objective visualization in the ontologization of FMS, the process is not complete. Specific etiology is still the ultimate rarefactive trump card in disease calibration. And while there is increasingly suggestive pathological data, a definitive etiology remains somewhat elusive. Almost every medical journal article I surveyed included a perfunctory statement acknowledging the lack of etiological understanding concerning FMS. The following excerpt from the journal *Arthritis and Rheumatism* is a fairly typical example:

> The etiology and pathogenesis of FMS are not well understood, but they are probably multifactorial. Available evidence points toward dysregulation of neurotransmitter function and central pain sensitization as fundamental mechanisms. (Crofford et al., 2005, pp. 1264–1265)

Many articles also describe the problems associated with treating a disease that is so little understood. Indeed, there is a great deal of concern about what constitutes "meaningful" treatment, as can be seen from the following excerpt:

> There is a lack of consensus about the definition of clinically meaningful reduction in pain for fibromyalgia clinical trials. In addition, it is unclear whether improvement in pain intensity alone should define response to treatment in fibromyalgia, which is a syndrome characterized by multiple symptoms in addition to pain. (Arnold, 2006, p. 220)

All in all, this debate over the ontology of FMS has created an environment of epistemological uncertainty among pain-management and FMS clinicians.

In figure 5.2, I have modified Latour's general diagram to demonstrate the constitutive CBD of FMS. As can be seen, the FMS pathologist is not able to identify a clear, specific etiology under the traditional rheumatologic model of FMS. There is no musculoskeletal evidence that would provide the foundation for an articulable specific etiology. This paucity of evidence causes an interruption in the pathological goals of documentation and subsequent treatment. Pathologists are then forced to detour through other disciplines to begin to articulate a specific etiology.

Again, the 1990 ACR diagnostic criteria operationalized a new mode of FMS inquiry. It detoured FMS from rheumatology to neurology and opened up new horizon of possibility in neuroimaging. The neuroimages themselves provided a new evidence base for pathological inquiry. As the following passage from *Chemist and Druggist* notes:

> Many clinicians traditionally regarded fibromyalgia as predominately psychosomatic, rather than neurological or physiological. However, advances over

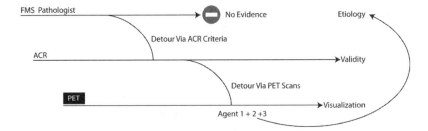

FIGURE 5.2. Detour and enrollment in the legitimization of FMS. When confronted with a lack of pathological evidence, FMS clinicians detour through the 1990 ACR criteria, and again through the neuroimaging black box. Of particular note is the detour through diagnostics and visualization in the establishment of a provisional etiology.

recent years might be on the verge of resolving these pathophysiological and therapeutic enigmas. For example, imaging studies reveal several differences in the brains of people with fibromyalgia compared to controls. ("Pharmacy Update," 2007, p. 17)

The detour through neuroimaging provides a benchmark for understanding the physiological differences between fibromyalgia patients and a healthy control group. These differences hint at a specific etiology grounded in the neurochemistry of pain processing. Indeed, the extended discussion from the aforementioned *Arthritis Research and Therapy* article outlines some of the initial evidence for CNS pain-processing irregularities:

At the present time, functional brain imaging in FMS has revealed the following insights. First, FMS patients differ from healthy controls in baseline levels of neural activity, specifically in the caudate nucleus. Second, administration of a noxious pressure or heat stimulus results in changes in brain activity consistent with verbal reports of patients' pain intensity. Third, like healthy controls, FMS patients normally detect and experience a full range of perceived pain magnitude; but sensations become unpleasant at stimulus intensity that are significantly lower than those observed in health controls. (Williams & Gracely, 2006, p. 230)

Obviously, this account of the ontologization of FMS harkens back to the PR / WT identified in the previous section. The traditional rejection of the legitimacy and reality of FMS could be understood as resulting from the institutions exercising their principles of PR / WT. Without identifiable markers of FMS, neither pathology nor diagnostics could make acceptable claims concerning FMS's reality. With the cause a mystery, specific etiology would not allow for pathological discussion of FMS. Similarly, without a statistically valid diagnostic criteria, the disorder could not even be differentiated from rheumatisms or mental illnesses. Of course, as the above narrative suggests, the establishment of a statistically valid diagnostic criteria—the 1990 ACR criteria—and the influence of PET data both paved the way for a pathological hypothesis (CNS dysregulation) and ontologization.

The fact that both the regulation of the sinus headache and the agency of FMS made use of these same PR / WT speaks as much to the relationship between constitutive and rarefactive calibration as it does to the affinity among different disease discourses. Specific etiology, diagnostic validity, and objective visualization are each readily available argumentative resources, whether the goal is constitution or rarefaction. Furthermore, these cases serve to reinforce my arguments about the importance of calibrating metadiscourse in the study of medical practice.

CHAPTER SIX

Networks of Calibration

Now, suppose you're an outfit called HelthWyzer. Suppose you make your money out of drugs and procedures that cure sick people, or else—better—that make it impossible for them to get sick in the first place. . . . So, what are you going to need, sooner or later? More cures? After that. . . . After you've cured everything going? So, you'd need more sick people. Or else—and it might be the same thing—more diseases. New and different ones. Right? Stands to reason . . . but don't they keep discovering new diseases? Not discovering . . . they're creating them. —Margaret Atwood, *Oryx and Crake*

Dystopian science fiction typically functions as a reification of techno-logical, scientific, and/or economic issues in contemporary culture, creating a vision of a future where the most disturbing and dangerous elements of our cultural landscape come to dominate. Margaret Atwood's *Oryx and Crake* (excerpted above) offers a compelling yet disturbing picture of a not-too-distant-future, a post-apocalyptic dystopia where nearly all humans have been wiped out by a deadly hemorrhagic virus. Atwood's narrative comprises two alternating timelines, one in the novel's present, and one in flashback—which details the events leading up to the end of humanity. The uncanny flashback narrative portrays contemporary cultural institutions reified and extruded into an ultimately pessimistic but not inconceivable vision of our near future. The centerpiece of the flash-back is the "compound"—the combination corporate campus/gated community where the intellectual elite have holed up to escape the violence and disease of the rest of society, the "pleeblands." The compounds are owned and operated by multinational pharmaceutical conglomerates that seem to have taken on a whole host of traditionally governmental responsibilities—including education, law enforcement, and military intelligence. What is perhaps most disturbing about Atwood's vision of this potential future is not the power that the pharmaceutical corporations exert over the personnel within the compounds, but the power they exert over the pleeblands—for it is these very companies that ultimately pave the way for the impending apocalypse.

Of the many problems associated with pharmaceutical corporations as reified in Atwood's compounds, this chapter is particularly concerned with the contemporary efforts to generate new market niches for their products. In Atwood's (2003) novel, these market niches are created through a combination of "problematics"—a communications field borne of a synthesis of "Applied Logic, Applied Rhetoric, Medical Ethics and Terminology, Applied Semantics, Relativistics and Advanced Mischaracterizations, Comparative Cultural Psychology" (p. 188), and intentional infection. While I do not think Atwood is suggesting that contemporary pharmaceutical companies are actually launching biological weapons, there is much in the way of critical studies of medicine that suggests they are involved in something that may amount to the same thing—infection via re-signification. That is, the marketing arm of pharmaceutical corporations sometimes takes typical moments of human discomfort, of dis-ease, and rebrands them as disease. The mechanisms through which dis-ease becomes disease are equally well explored in Atwood's novel, but through the lens of its protagonist narrator, Jimmy/Snowman, who becomes one of these marketing gurus:

> Cosmetic creams, workout equipment, Joltbars to build your muscle-scape into a breathtaking marvel of sculpted granite. Pills to make you fatter, thinner, hairier, balder, whiter, browner, blacker, yellower, sexier, and happier. It was his task to describe and extol, to present the vision of what—oh, so easily!—could come to be. Hope and fear, desire and revulsion, these were his stocks-in-trade, on these he rang his changes. (p. 248)

Here we see a description of a noncalibrating form of ontological constitution. Atwood portrays a model of health and medical marketing where pharmaceutical and supplement manufacturers simply evoke new ontologies by fiat. New diseases are simply called into being through marketing and for the benefit for shareholders and the corporate bottom line.

I start with Atwood's dystopian speculative fiction because it serves as an excellent avatar of postmodern and critical-cultural studies of health and medicine and their tacit commission of the hegemonic fallacy. In so doing, this research, owing a strong debt to neo-Marxist thought and critical-cultural theory, presents a dystopian worldview where an all-powerful Big

Pharma runs roughshod over disempowered consumers within a laby-rinthine and unwieldy medical-industrial complex (MIC). For example, much work in bioethics and critical-cultural studies of medicine offers ac-counts of how the marketing arms of Big Pharma have medicalized the manifold discomforts of the human experience. Work in this area often focuses on the so-called practices of pharmaco-psychiatry, which stage lower-limb fidgets as restless leg syndrome (Woloshin & Schwartz, 2006; Moynihan & Henry, 2006; Williams, Martin & Gabe, 2011), shyness as social anxiety disorder/agoraphobia (Moynihan, Heath & Henry, 2002; Wolinsky, 2005; Rose, 2006), and sadness as neurotransmitter imbalances (Lewis, 2003; Gardner, 2003; Healy, 2004).

Certainly, pharmaceutical corporations have been responsible for more than their fair share of misery in the forms of price gouging (Cle-land, 2004; Angell, 2005) and ghost authorship of clinical trials (Sismondo, 2007; Gøtzsche, Hróbjartsson, Johansen, Haahr, Altman & Chan, 2007; Elliott, 2010), as well as conducting predatory clinical trials in third-world countries (Glickman, McHutchison, Peterson, Cairns, Harrington, Califf & Schulman, 2009; Annas, 2009; Petryna, 2009), and even publishing fake, seemingly scientific journals offering supposedly independent analyses of their products (Hutson, 2009; Moynihan, 2009). And certainly, as my ex-ploration of the case of the sinus headache suggests, pharmaceutical com-panies have also inappropriately propagated cures for diseases of dubious legitimacy. Nevertheless, I would argue that the work of the previous chapter on principles of rarefaction as warranting topoi demonstrate at least a strong possibility that institutions of rarefaction ranging from med-ical disciplines to federal regulatory agencies are capable of providing some checks on the supposedly unlimited power of Big Pharma to stage dis-ease as disease.

Subsequently, this chapter is devoted to exploring the role of phar-maceutical companies and federal regulatory agencies in rarefactive and constitutive calibration. Until this point, I have been exploring ontologi-cal calibration primarily through the practices of the three institutions of rarefaction explored in detail in the last chapter—the scientific disci-plines of pathology, diagnostics, and radiology. In contrast, the work of this chapter traces the practices of rarefactive and constitutive calibration into the intersectional networks of the MIC. Here I will continue to use *MIC* as a convenient shorthand for the complex intersections of pharma-ceutics, medical disciplines, and regulatory agencies. However, I do not intend the term in the monolithic, all-powerful sense often deployed by critical-cultural theorists. Rather, I use it quite simply to refer to the network, the assemblage, the interactional matrix of institutions of rarefaction involved in calibrating disease.

Ultimately, I'll make the case that the MIC as a network of calibration is much more difficult to navigate than invocations of the hegemonic fallacy vis-à-vis Big Pharma would suggest. In so doing, I will first offer a brief exegesis of the hegemonic fallacy in critical-cultural studies of pharmaceuticals and then unpack the dense calibrating networks that surround the FDA's mission of rarefactive oversight. Subsequently, I will revisit the cases of the sinus headache and FMS as the ontological debates are taken up beyond the cross-disciplinary deliberation and into the policy arena. As these cases will demonstrate, different calibrating efforts activate different pathways in the calibrating networks of the MIC. Such differential activations challenge the notion of an impenetrable MIC run by Big Pharma. While not all calibrating efforts end in a victory for consumers, I will still argue that the opportunities for beneficial outcomes serve to demonstrate the failure of the hegemonic model for investigating contemporary pharmaceuticals and the regulatory landscape that surrounds it.

The Hegemonic Fallacy in Critical Studies of Medicine

The opening excerpt is one of the moments in *Oryx and Crake* where the fiction is uncannily close to the actual work of critical-cultural studies of medicine. Indeed, many have argued that the marketing arm of the pharmaceutical industry is responsible for the proliferation of certain diseases that capitalize on what, in a prior era, might just have been considered the normal (albeit unpleasant) side of human existence. For some time now, medical humanists and medical ethicists have been exploring the role of the pharmaceutical industry in the creation/legitimization/propagation of new illnesses. This exploration has largely focused on the relationship between the pharmaceutical industry and psychiatry/biopsychiatry. These critical analyses often focus on the articulations among diagnostic categories (often represented by the *Diagnostic and Statistical Manual of Mental Illness [DSM]*), pharmaceutical advertising, and third-party reimbursement practices (Gardner, 2003; Aho, 2008; Elliott, 2003). Echoing Atwood's critique, Elliott argues that the pharmaceutical industry has intentionally engaged in the production of disease. Of course, rather than the actual production of a harmful biological agent, this is disease creation through re-signification, through what Atwood dubs "problematics"—that is, through marketing: "At least part of what has happened is the marketing of a disease," contends Elliott in *Better Than Well* (2003, p. 124). Similarly, in the case of antidepressants, Gardner notes that "antidepressant marketing schemes sell the idea that depression is an illness, antidepressants work, while authorizing the larger depression script" (2003, p. 124). Indeed, Elliott's characterization of pharmaceuticals and Atwood's description of compound problematics parallel each other almost perfectly:

> Within this framework, suffering becomes a problem of brain chemistry. A drug that fixes the chemistry solves the problem of suffering. Death, loss, grief, fear, anxiety, sexual inadequacy become medical problems to be addressed by experts with prescription pads. Thus do the existential interests of a moral being harmonize perfectly, in a way that only Adam Smith could appreciate, with the financial interests of the pharmaceutical industry. (2003, pp. 157–158)

And as Aho also notes, the same process is evident in scientific publications for contemporary ailments such as the *DSM*:

> With the *DSM*'s rapidly expanding number of diagnostic categories and new medications being introduced to treat them, everyday emotional suffering and behavior—such as worrying, anger, frustration, restlessness, even the inability to get an erection—can now be medicalized as biological diseases that can be treated with a particular drug. (p. 244)

In fact (according to the research of Elliott, Aho, Gardner, and many others), the integration of pharmaceutical marketing and practical/scientific literature is so complete that it is often difficult to differentiate one from the other.

As Elliott describes it, "The genius of much of today's pharmaceutical marketing is that it does not look like marketing at all. Very often, it looks like science" (pp. 124–125). Gardner, in his criticism of antidepressant research and advertising, also highlights the links between science and marketing:

> Overzealous drug use and promotion, then, is due not only to pharmaceutical company influence, but to the repetitive biopsychiatric script that floats contradictory research findings, reifies the single cause model, and recognizes antidepressant drugs as the route to a (near) cure. Contradictory claims praising

and critiquing antidepressants are largely nonexistent in consumer literature, encouraging public confidence and ongoing research monies. The constrained discourse translates easily into marketing schemes. (p. 124)

All these (often valid) concerns over the relationships between psychiatry, medicine, and the pharmaceutical industry have led to sometimes scathing criticism by medical humanists and medical ethicists. These critiques often paint a hegemonic picture rather like Atwood's dystopian vision wherein dark cabals of pharmaceutical executives are mercilessly profiting on the naïveté of the unwitting medical consumer.

Similarly, as Lewis (2003) describes it, psychotherapy is built on a foundation of hidden ideological forces that configure practice and treatment:

> Psychotherapy, no different from psychopharmacologic technoscience, is also intertwined in political forces that are rarely articulated and critiqued within the psychotherapy discourse community. Perhaps the only thing one could say in favor of psychotherapy is that, compared to biopsychiatry, the earlier era of psychotherapeutic psychiatry was not backed by a major bioscience industry and a new breed of corporate medicine. (p. 57)

This hegemony of pharmacological medicine tightly constrains both consumer choice and the possibility of consumer criticism, or as Gardner clarifies, "the good consumer-citizen is expected to passively embrace the link between mental health technologies of surveillance and treatment, accept biotechnologies as the *solution* to productivity lapses, and to leave the critique to the policy of science experts" (p. 126).

While I have deep concerns about this portrayal of pharmacological medical science, it's important to note that critical scholars of medicine are not always entirely beholden to a hegemonic vision of the MIC. Indeed, my exploration of the interactional calibrating matrix of the MIC mirrors an area of inquiry opened up by Carl Elliott's *Better Than Well* (2003). With the luxury of a book-length text, Elliott is able to temper his criticism not so much of the pharmaceutical industry but of the healthcare providers and researchers who are constrained nearly as much as the patients. Even though pharmaceutical marketing has a tendency to sell illness as much as treatment, he acknowledges:

> *This does not mean that drug companies are simply making up diseases out of thin air*, or the psychiatrists are being gulled into diagnosing well people as

sick. No one doubts that some people generally suffer from, say, depression, or attention-deficit/hyperactivity disorder, or that the right medications make these disorders better. But surrounding the core of many of these disorders is a wide zone of ambiguity that can be chiseled out and expanded. Pharmaceutical companies have powerful financial interest in expanding categories of mental disease, because *it is only when a certain condition is recognized as a disease that it can be treated with the products that the companies produce.* The bigger the diagnostic category, the more patients who will fit within its boundaries, and the more psychoactive drugs they will be prescribed. (p. 124, emphasis added)

Here, I want to echo Elliott's acknowledgment. Given the density of articulations that make up the MIC, it seems unlikely, as Elliott suggests, that any individual pharmaceutical organization could simply declare that a new disease exists now simply because they've developed a new drug to peddle. This suggests strongly to me that the rarefactive and calibrating forces of various institutions of rarefaction within the MIC are capable of, at least at times, challenging the will of Big Pharma. As I've alluded to above, the FDA with its legally granted authority occupies a pivotal position at the center of the MIC and subsequently can activate calibrating and rarefying assemblages as it adjudicates the efforts of pharmaceutical corporations. It is these assemblage activations I will trace in the next sections.

The FDA's Network of Calibration

As noted in the last chapter, when the FDA *indicates* that a drug is safe and effective for treating a given disease, such a declaration can provide legitimacy for both a drug and the disease it treats. "Indication" is a technical-regulatory term here. FDA approval means a new drug is approved for the treatment of a given condition. The drug is then said to be indicated for that disease. Drug indications follow years (and sometimes decades) of coordinated work at the intersections among multiple regimes of practical engagement, institutions of rarefaction—each with its own principles of rarefaction and mechanisms of calibration. For example, FDA indications are typically based on the results of RCTs published in scholarly journals (empirical-discursive ontology), under the oversight of editors and peer-review boards (institutions of rarefaction). The publication of an RCT typically requires as part of its methodology section a clearly described and statistically valid means of identifying trial subjects—valid diagnostic criteria (principle or rarefaction), which, as I explained in the previous chapter, is typically knit with pathological evidence (principle of rarefaction). Subsequently, a typical FDA indication requires that the discourse of the pharmaceutical label be rarefied and legitimized by the principles of rarefaction deployed by diagnostics, pathology, pharmacy, and the regulatory offices of the FDA.

The authority for the FDA's rarefactive and calibrating practices are grounded in the Federal Food, Drug, and Cosmetic Act. While this law provides the foundation for oversight and regulation of many products including human food, animal feed, medical instruments, and cosmetics, it is section 505 that is particularly relevant to the question of new diseases and drugs:

> No person shall introduce or deliver for introduction into interstate commerce any new drug, unless an approval of an application filed pursuant to subsection (b) or (j) is effective with respect to such drug.

Subsections (b) and (j) are those that require would-be pharmaceutical vendors to demonstrate safety and efficacy through legitimized research practices. The primary mechanism of this research oversight is the FDA's Center for Drug Evaluation and Research (CDER, pronounced "cedar"). Under the oversight of CDER, the primary mechanism of preapproval testing is the RCT. As CDER notes on its website:

> Clinical trials represent the ultimate premarket testing ground for unapproved drugs. During these trials, an investigation compound is administered to humans and is evaluated for its safety and effectiveness in treating, preventing, or diagnosing a specific disease or condition. The results of this testing will comprise the single most important factor in the approval or disapproval of a new drug. (Food and Drug Administration, 2009)

However, one RCT is never sufficient for drug approval. In fact, several trials are rarely adequate. CDER outlines a four-phase process for pharmaceutical research and evaluation, the first three of which are required before any new drug can be marketed or sold. As suggested in the above quote, these phases evaluate the safety and efficacy of new drugs. Each phase of research is regulated by a combination of CDER's scientific and ethical standards designed both to elicit appropriate safety and efficacy data and to safeguard study participants' rights and safety. Fig-

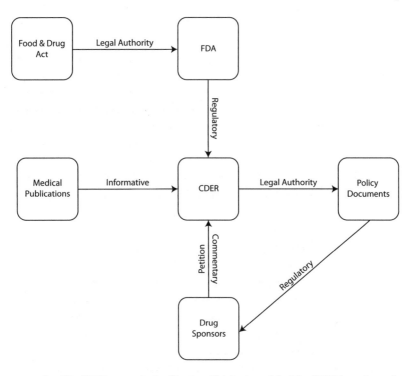

FIGURE 6.1. The FDA's network of calibration. This basic model of the CDER's work to calibrate disease ontologies and regulate (rarefy) disease discourse highlights the legal authority of the FDA to regulate the pharmaceuticals industry and the stipulated role of medical publications to inform CDER's regulatory activity.

ure 6.1 provides a sketch of the basic framework for the FDA's network of calibration.

While drug approval studies are designed to meet the standards outlined by CDER, they are also subject to additional regulation/regularization. The research reports following RCTs typically find their way into the peer-reviewed scholarly journals of medicine and pharmacology. And as would be expected, the research protocols are subject to the disciplinary standards of each journal and enforced through the mechanisms of editorial oversight and peer review. It is these standards that, perhaps, have the most effect in preventing the invention of disease. In order for an RCT to be considered valid and legitimate, it has to pair a diagnosable disease with a controllable intervention (drug). Diagnostics is its own subspecialty with its own disciplinary journals and subsequent regularizing influence. Diagnosis of a disorder now typically relies on what are called "validity studies"—studies that evaluate the statistical soundness of diagnostic criteria.

When a proposal for a new drug, or new use (indication) for an old drug, is presented to CDER for approval, a range of possible nodes and articulations can be activated. In the clearest of cases, cases where the evidence in favor of approval is overwhelming, new drugs or indications may be granted summary review and approval. However, for more complicated proposals, a different pathway is activated and the case is sent to the appropriate drug advisory committee, or DAC. CDER has established DACs in seventeen areas of clinical research, including oncology and hematology, rheumatology, psychopharmacology, antiviral therapy, gastroenterology, and nonprescription drugs. These committees are tasked with investigating and evaluating available evidence and making a policy recommendation for or against new drug or device approvals and indications. These investigations follow a modified judicial formation wherein drug sponsors offer an argumentative presentation in favor of drug approval, the FDA offers a counterpresentation, and both sides are cross-examined by the DAC members. It is not uncommon for DAC approval hearings to take four to eight hours to adjudicate a single case.

OTC medications, like most of those offered for the sinus headache, are regulated by the FDA in much the same way as prescription medications. Newly introduced drugs must undergo rigorous safety and efficacy studies. Actually, the safety requirements for OTC medications are even stricter, since they must be deemed safe enough to be self-administered. Most new medications added to the list of FDA-approved OTC medications are those that have been reclassified through the FDA Prescription-to-OTC program, another possible articulation that can be activated as part of calibrating and rarefactive practices. Once a drug is classified as OTC, FDA regulatory efforts shift to labeling concerns. That is, the FDA regulates what efficacy claims can be printed on the label as well as dosing information and safety warnings. Given this, patients and physicians are prone to trust the product statements offered by the various OTC medication providers.

Although my exegesis so far has focused primarily on sketching the FDA's network of calibration in terms of new drug approval, it should also be noted that the regulatory arm of FDA oversight also includes ongoing surveillance and enforcement activities. CDER monitors prescription and OTC packaging and products on the market in the United States to ensure that drugs are correctly labeled and formulated. In the cases of pharmaceutical error or willful violation, the FDA has the authority to inspect facilities, require changes to packages, issue mandatory recall orders, and even shut down companies, if need be. (Although such actions are much less common today, reading about the infancy of the FDA evokes Prohibition and Eliot Ness.) Additionally, the FDA has the authority to issue and enforce rule changes. This is a process I will describe in more detail in the case of the sinus headache. According to federal law, proposed rule changes must allow for public commentary. This is why two different possibilities for pharmaceutical-CDER communication (new drug/indication petitions and proposed rule commentary) are listed in figure 6.1.

Sinus Headaches

The case of sinus headaches provides an ideal entrée for my inquiry into the differential activations of networks of calibration that surround the FDA, especially regarding the potential for the FDA and CDER to challenge the supposed hegemony of Big Pharma. As I noted in the previous chapter's exploration of clinical studies of sinus headaches, many researchers and clinicians who doubt the validity of the sinus headache frame their contributions as a challenge to the power of industry and Madison Avenue. Indeed, if the efforts to reclassify most supposed sinus headache sufferers as migraineurs are successful, it will mean a significant potential loss of profit for manufacturers of OTC sinus headache medicines. The question that remains is to what extent the FDA will incorporate the new clinical understanding of "migraines presenting as sinus headaches" into their policy-making or enforcement practices.

As it turns out, there is some potential movement in this area. In 2004, the FDA took specific regulatory measures to address an incongruity between OTC sinus decongestant claims and the scientific understanding of sinusitis. Use and effect claims for such medications are governed primarily by the Code of Federal Regulations' *Cold, Cough, Allergy, Bronchodilator, and Antiasthmatic Drug Products for Over-the-Counter Human Use* (2014). This document was originally established in 1976 by the Advisory Review Panel on OTC Cold, Cough, Allergy, Bronchodilator and Antiasthmatic Drugs Products (henceforth, the Panel). This document identifies what specific language is allowed for efficacy claims for cold and cough OTC products. That is, it specifies a list of potentially eligible statements that can be placed on the back of a product's packaging. For example, it allows a drug (subject to approval for the specific active ingredient) to claim that it "temporarily relieves nasal congestion" or "temporarily relieves sinus congestion and pressure." The document further provides drug manufacturers with the option of appending specific disease claims to those effects statements. Subsequently, a drug claim statement might read "temporarily relieves nasal congestion due to hay fever." In the original 1976 document, one of the acceptable options for this secondary clause was "associated with sinusitis."

On August 2, 2004, the FDA issued a proposed rule change in the *Federal Register* that would strip this last clause from the list of eligible statements. Specifically, the proposed rule change argued, "The [1976] Panel did not provide any explanation for this indication in its general discussion of OTC nasal decongestants (41 FR 38312 at 38396 to 38397) or in its Category I labeling discussion" ("Cold, Cough, Allergy," 2004, p. 46119). In further justifying the proposed rule change, the FDA argued that new evidence had come to light casting doubt on the appropriateness of the "associated with sinusitis" clause:

> Recent publications (Refs. 1 and 2) indicate that prospective studies on the role of nasal decongestants in the treatment of sinusitis are lacking, and the data on their use as an adjunct in the treatment of sinusitis are limited and controversial. (p. 46120)

References 1 and 2 here are scholarly publications in the *Journal of Allergy and Clinical Immunology* and *Pediatrics* from 1998 and 2001, respectively. Their use here constitutes a clear example of calibration by enrollment. The FDA enrolls the scholarly literature into its calibrating program of action in order to warrant their objections to pharmaceuticals. The inclusion of these sources in the proposed rule changes highlights the influence of scholarly medical research on the regulatory process and confirms that such research does not have to support the interests of pharmaceutical companies in order to be incorporated into new regulations.

Proposed rule changes include a mandatory public comment period. Regulations.gov (the website that manages these comments) indicates that six comments were filed, but the final rule publication references only three comments. Of the three comments discussed in the final rule notice ("Cold, Cough, Allergy," 2005), one objected to the proposed rule change and two supported it. Although no information about the dissenting commenter was provided, it seems very likely that it was an OTC decongestant manufacturer. The supporting commenters were identified as the

American Academy of Allergy, Asthma & Immunology (AAAAI) and a "consumer." The FDA's recitation of the dissenting comment distilled the argument in a nine-point bulleted list that argued, among other things: (1) The proposed rule change underestimates the health savvy of OTC decongestant consumers; (2) the proposed rule change is not based on sufficient or credible scientific evidence; and (3) the proposed rule change is not supported by guidelines from physician organizations. This last argument was rather quickly rebuffed, as one of the primary referenced set of guidelines was provided by the AAAAI. The other two primary arguments were rejected based on evidentiary grounds. In the first case, the FDA rejected the argument based on the commenter's failure to provide evidence that consumers would not be confused or misled. In the second case, the FDA asserted that the scholarly consensus was that there was no evidence to support the use of OTC decongestants for the treatment of sinusitis. After the mandatory comment period, the proposed rule was enacted on October 11, 2005, and OTC decongestant manufacturers were subsequently prohibited from making any claims about the use of their products for patients with sinusitis. This is why I argue that the hegemonic fallacy and its construal of an all-powerful Big Pharma leads scholars astray. The FDA, at least in this case, rejected the interests (and possibly the direct arguments) of pharmaceutical manufacturers in favor of efficacy data and public safety.

This analysis of the FDA deliberation regarding the sinusitis rule change allows for a more nuanced understanding of the rarefactive network that surrounds OTC drugs policy. Professional organizations and scholarly publications are tightly entangled in the network of calibration providing additional avenues wherein the hegemony of industry may be challenged. Figure 6.2 elaborates figure 6.1 and accounts for this expanded understanding of the FDA's calibrating assemblage.

Furthermore, this brief analysis demonstrates the FDA exercise rarefactive calibration across the diverse nodes of the MIC. The vehicle of the *Federal Register* allows for the issuances of a proposed rule changes, while Regulations.gov allows commentary. And the *Federal Register* again serves as a venue for rebuttal and decision making. In this case, the FDA adjudicators performed a rarefactive calibration among the various ontologies staged by the marketing practices of pharmaceuticals, the OTC practices of suffering consumers, the empirical-discursive practices of medical research, and the clinical practices of otolaryngologists as codified in the AAAAI comment. The final rule publication presents a variant of adding up; the differential comments were tabulated: one against, two

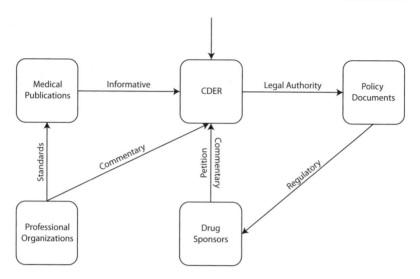

FIGURE 6.2. FDA rule revision network of calibration. This elaboration of figure 6.1 offers a more complete accounting of the network articulations activated in the proposed rule revision for OTC cold medications and sinusitis. The articulation density surrounding medical publications and professional organizations helps provide CDER's regulatory program of action with sufficient power to limit the work of the pharmaceutical industry.

in favor. This adding up is further buttressed by rarefactive calibration by linking the empirical-discursive research to the AAAAI practice and thus overturning the interests of OTC manufacturers.

Now, it should not go without noting that this rule change has not yet fully curtailed the efforts of sinus headache medicine manufacturers. As with most such completed issues, there is an additional regulatory wrinkle. The 2005 rule change specifically impacted drug claims. "Drug claims" is a very specific technical term for the box (typically on the back of the package) labeled "uses." This is the difficulty for sinus headache medication. A representative example can be found on the label for Sudafed Sinus Headache. The "uses" section lists the following as derived from the new final monograph for cold and cough medicine:

- Temporarily relieves headache, minor aches, and pains
- Temporarily relieves nasal congestion

As per FDA guidelines, there are no claims related to sinusitis. The product does not explicitly claim to treat sinus headache. Rather, it is named "Sinus Headache™."

As previously mentioned, the new final monograph rule explicitly targets the "uses" section. It does specifically impact a product's trade name (or in FDA parlance, proprietary name). This, however, does not mean that the FDA is powerless to address sinus headache medicines should it choose to do so. In this case, two different calibrating articulations can be activated. Jurisdiction for proprietary names regulation is divided between CDER's Divisions of Drug Marketing, Advertising, and Communications as well as Medication Error Prevention and Analysis. A bifurcated review process subjects newly proprietary names to evaluation for (1) the potential to mislead customers and (2) the potential to cause clinician or pharmacy confusion. It is this first "promotional review" that is of primary concern here. According to the FDA (n.d.) guidance document:

> CDER's Division of Drug Marketing, Advertising, and Communications (DDMAC) evaluates proposed proprietary names to determine if they are overly fanciful, so as to misleadingly imply unique effectiveness or composition, as well as to assess whether they contribute to overstatement of product efficacy, minimization of risk, broadening of product indications, or making of unsubstantiated superiority claims. (p. 2)

This policy provides the regulatory framework to adjudicate promotional names in the case of potentially misleading claims. Subsequently, a company like Bayer Pharmaceuticals cannot simply rebrand one of their aspirin products as Bayer CuresCancer™ just to sell more boxes. Doing so would violate FDA propriety names policy and activate rarefactive activities by the DDMAC and the Division of Medical Error.

Therefore, it would seem to be a simple matter of policy enforcement to restrict products with the name "sinus headache" from being marketed in the United States. At the time of this writing, this has not yet happened. Part of the reason for this is no doubt institutional. Promotional name review primarily takes place as part of the new drug approval process. The "sinus headache" name has been long approved by the FDA, and its approval was consistent with the scientific understanding at the time of its approval. Certainly, the 2005 sinusitis revision cites evidence published in 1998 and 2001. Perhaps a certain amount of lag time is necessary between the establishment of a new scientific consensus and a change in regulatory policy or enforcement actions.

Before I transition to my inquiry into FMS regulation, there is one more avenue of analysis that cannot be ignored in my discussion of sinus headaches. To simply say that the scholarly and clinical work rejecting the

sinus headache challenges the hegemony of Big Pharma because it cur-
tails the purchasing of OTC sinus headache medication ignores broader
impacts of such a rejection. The ontology of sinus headaches is not simply rejected. No one claims that sinus headache sufferers are not suffering. Rather, it is claimed that the activity of "sinus headache" sufferers
actually stages an ontology of migraines. Such a re-diagnosis shifts the
location and form of treatment for these patients. They are no longer
self-medicating or seeing GPs or, in severe cases, otolaryngologists. As
migraine patients, they must see neurologists. (And here we see again
the neuroimperialism discussed in chapter 4.) Correspondingly, these
patients no longer take relatively inexpensive OTC analgesics or decongestants. Instead, they are prescribed much more expensive migraine
medicines such as triptans. Even in cases where relatively inexpensive generic medications are prescribed, the added costs of visiting a neurologist
make treatment for migraines far more expensive than treatment for sinus
headaches. It is also worth noting that of the clinical studies cited in the
last chapter, many of the authors are neurologists or headache specialists
and stand to benefit greatly from shifting "sinus headache" patients from
otolaryngology to neurology. While only two of the cited studies disclosed
funding sources, those sources were GlaxoSmithKline and Ortho-McNeil,
manufacturers of prescription migraine drugs Imitrex and Topomax, respectively. (Although it should be noted that Ortho-McNeil also manu-
factures a number of sinus headache drugs, including Sudafed.) Indeed,
any hasty Internet search will find that GlaxoSmithKline has sponsored a
great number of studies, conferences, and educational seminars devoted
to re-diagnosing sinus headache patients and migraineurs. Ultimately, this
subsequent analysis provides us with an even more complicated model of
the various influences on federal drugs policy (see figure 6.3).

   This last avenue of analysis leaves me with a certain aporia regarding
how effectively the FDA leverages its place at the center of the MIC to
contest the hegemony of Big Pharma. On the one hand, otolaryngology
and neurology researchers have both contributed significantly to rede-
fining sinus headache. This work seems to be both of potential benefit
for patients (better diagnosis) and of negative benefit to pharmaceutical
manufacturers (fewer inappropriate products sold). On the other hand,
the shifting of so many patients from otolaryngology to neurology and
from inexpensive OTC medications to expensive prescription medications potentially confirms our worst fears about the MIC. I wish I could
offer an easy verdict here, but the complexity and ongoing nature of the
sinus headache debates means I must continue to withhold judgment.

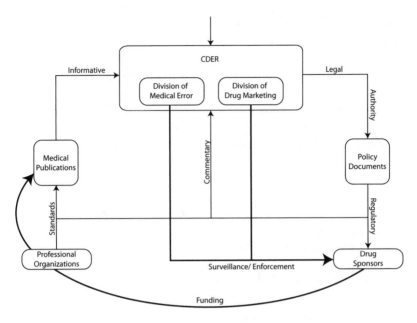

FIGURE 6.3. Proprietary name regulation and pharmaceuticals funding. This network model provides an even further elaboration to figure 6.1, extending figure 6.2's documentation of the role of medical publications and professional organizations in pharmaceutical regulation. Specifically, it highlights the funding relationship between industry and medical research that may potentially contravene the regulatory and surveillance efforts of CDER.

Fibromyalgia

FMS provides a second and equally vexing case of FDA regulation and that regulation's relationship with pharmaceutical manufacturers. Addressing the morality of the ontologization of FMS is a fraught issue. Millions of predominantly female patients were being denied adequate care because their illness was unrecognized by the mainstream medical establishment. The ontologization of FMS and the subsequent approval of Lyrica had a very positive impact on the preexisting lack of treatment options for fibromyalgics. And yet, potentially millions of patients are now purchasing Lyrica, an expense that did not exist before. Indeed, a recent Institute of Medicine (2009) report on conflict of interest in health education, research, and policy singles out a patient advocacy group, the National Fibromyalgia Association (NFA), for receiving upward of 40 percent of its funding from pharmaceutical manufacturers (p. 220). Furthermore, Kristin Barker, in a 2011 article in *Social Science & Medicine,* persuasively declares the alliance between Pfizer and the NFA an act of "pharmaceuticals opportunism" (p. 836):

> Increasing public awareness of fibromyalgia and declaring its status as "real" have been major prongs in Pfizer's plan to capitalize on the fibromyalgia market. In August 2007 Pfizer joined forces with the largest fibromyalgia advocacy organization in the United States, the National Fibromyalgia Association (NFA), to create a fibromyalgia awareness campaign. The Pfizer-NFA campaign included a televised public service announcement and an interactive website. (p. 836)

The complexity of relations among various entities including CDER, the relevant DAC (the Arthritis Advisory Committee, or AAC), the NFA, and pharmaceutical companies provides a very difficult arena in which to adjudicate the impacts of conflicts of interest and industry funding on the regulatory process. To demonstrate the complexity of this issue, I will trace Lyrica's path to approval, highlighting along the way all the players in the densely tangled calibrating network that was activated during this process.

As previously noted, Lyrica was the first drug approved in the United States specifically for the treatment of FMS. In this case, the request was for a new indication: Lyrica was already approved for the treatment of neuropathic pain associated with diabetic peripheral neuropathy and postherpetic neuralgia epilepsy, and it was subsequently indicated in the treatment of epilepsy and seizure disorders. The new indication for FMS application was submitted on December 20, 2006, and approval was issued on June 6, 2007. Due to the prior history of Lyrica's approval—which indicates documented safety and efficacy for related pain conditions—the new indication for FMS appears to have been perfunctory. Additionally, the new Lyrica indication for FMS was subject to priority review as, according to the review documents, "fibromyalgia is a serious condition for which there are no approved drug products to date" (FDA Center for Drug Evaluation and Research, 2007, p. 2). In total, the indication took six months from application to the issuance of the final approval letter (Department of Health and Human Services, n.d.), which includes no demands for additional postmarket studies in the primary patient, although it does require follow-up studies on pediatric patients.

Interestingly, the approval documents for the Lyrica indication do not hedge about the reality of FMS. It is presented straightforwardly as a recognized illness, albeit one with a little-understood etiology. Of course, as was the case with the journal literature discussed in chapter 4, the availability of neuroimaging data is presented to offset this lack of understanding:

> Fibromyalgia is a syndrome characterized by chronic diffuse musculoskeletal pain, disordered sleep and fatigue that is frequently associated with a variety of nonspecific complaints such as cognitive difficulties, depression, anxiety, and headaches. . . . The etiology of fibromyalgia has not been currently identified but it is thought to be related to aberrancies in the central nervous system as manifested by functional MRI scans in patients with this disease associated with abnormal pain processing. (Neuner, 2007, p. 7)

In many ways, the clear and direct nature of this ontological proclamation and the relative ease of the indication approval were made possible by prior work at the AAC.

The AAC as node in the calibrating assemblages of the FDA was activated and convened a special meeting on June 23, 2003, specifically to address FMS. Indeed, the importance of this meeting for establishing the review criteria under which Lyrica would be evaluated was cited explicitly in the Lyrica indication review document (FDA Center for Drug Evaluation and Research, 2007, pp. 2, 8). Most DAC meetings center around the adjudication of new drug proposals. That is, pharmaceutical manufacturers submit the results of safety and efficacy trials as part of their efforts to demonstrate the scientific foundation for a new drug and to secure FDA approval. However, periodically, DACs will take up additional topics related to their primary subspecialties. In this case, the AAC met to develop a possible framework for making a claim for drugs that treat FMS. This procedure is, in this case at least, the prescription drug equivalent to the OTC regulation debates surrounding sinusitis. When a sinus decongestant is approved, drug marketers can choose claims like "relieves sinus congestion and pressure," and they used to be able to select "associated with sinusitis." In short, the purpose of the special AAC meeting was to develop possible acceptable grounds on which the claim "for the management of fibromyalgia" could be made.

While the calibrating efforts of the FDA have many opportunities to activate different nodes and bring different institutions of rarefaction into the current assemblage, it is important to note that pharmaceutical companies can also activate network pathways for their benefit. As the hegemonic critiques of Big Pharma anticipate, these pathway activations are typically accomplished via money. DACs present pharmaceutical companies with a unique opportunity to enroll more nodes in their program of action. While regular FDA employees are subject to strict prohibitions over financial relationships with industry, the special government employees (SGEs) that serve on DACs have a little more leeway (Crimes and Criminal Procedure, 2014). DAC SGEs who are employed by, receive speaker fees from, or have research funding by the pharmaceutical companies petitioning CDER may, if they are deemed to have essential expertise for the specific matter, be granted a conflict-of-interest waiver (FDA, 2008).

Like most DAC meetings, the special AAC gathering involved a collection of standing committee members, consultants for the current meeting, an industry representative, a patient representative (in this case the founder and president of the NFA), and members of the FDA staff. Following standard DAC procedures, the consultants were divided into voting and nonvoting members based on financial industry relationships. So for example, the industry representative and those consultants affiliated with pharmaceutical companies involved in FMS clinical trials were designated nonvoting. Now we see the FDA activating another network pathway, conflict-of-interest policies, so as to limit undue influence from Big Pharma. Pharmaceutical companies can fund some DAC members, with certain limits placed on their participation. However, in the case of the AAC meeting on FMS, this stratification of participation meant a lot less than it typically does. When a drug sponsor petitions a DAC for new drug approval, the meeting ends with a vote for or against approval. Nonvoting members, as one would expect, cannot participate. But since there was no proposal before the special AAC meeting, there was no vote. Thus, designating some members "nonvoting" was largely a meaningless effort.

Typically, in accordance with FDA guidelines, conflicts of interest are disclosed at the start of each meeting. The AAC meeting was no different. However, it was unique in the number of conflict waivers that were issued:

> In accordance with 18 United States Code, section 208(b)(3), the Food and Drug Administration has granted waivers for the following individuals, because the agency has determined that the need for their services outweighs the potential for conflict of interest. They include Gary Firestein, Dr. Gary Hoffman, Dr. Steven Abramson, Dr. Allan Gibofsky, Dr. Dennis Turk, Dr. Nathaniel Katz, and Dr. Laurence Bradley. (Food and Drug Administration, 2003, pp. 9–10)

This is, of course, the entire list of designated voting consultants. An additional partial waiver was issued to nonvoting consultant Dr. Daniel Clauw, who was allowed to give one expert presentation but then was required to remain silent for the remainder of the meeting. Dr. Leslie Crofford (guest speaker) and Dr. Fred Lasky (industry representative from Genzyme Diagnostics) were the only formal participants required to disclose their industry ties. At one point during the meeting, an audience member (Dr. Vibeke Strand) asked a question of one of the presenters. Again following FDA guidelines, she was required to disclose her conflicts of interest. When she promised to e-mail them in later rather than disclose them aloud, meeting moderator Dr. Cary Firestein declared that no further questions would be taken from audience members so as to avoid the hassles of reporting requirements.

Although we know from Barker's article and the Institute of Medicine report that the NFA has strong financial support from Pfizer, the patient representative declared no conflict of interest. For the purposes of DAC meetings, patient representatives are also designated SGEs and reimbursed for their time (FDA, 2010). As such, they are subject to conflict-of-interest polices. While there is no evidence to indicate (nor do I believe) that the patient representative was intentionally engaging in any sort of unethical or malicious behavior, this does raise some concerns. Further research into FDA conflict of interest and DACs should investigate the extent of potential patient representative conflicts and how frequently those conflicts are disclosed. It would not surprise me to learn that such disclosures are frequently glossed over. In the DAC meetings I have studied (both as a part of this project and others), ongoing rarefactive calibration typically elides the patient representative, marking it as "unscientific" and "anecdotal." Such a view likely encourages the notion that disclosure is not necessary since patient representative contributions lack the presumption of unscrupulous credibility held for the impartial scientist.

The patient representative and the industry representative did not participate as much as the other committee members and guest speakers. The industry representative was not given the opportunity to offer a formal presentation, and the patient representative's presentation was much shorter than any of the others. Additionally, neither participated to any great extent in the question-and-answer sessions nor in the discussion portions of the meeting. Nevertheless, each company with relationships to these speakers had or has a strong vested interest in the outcome

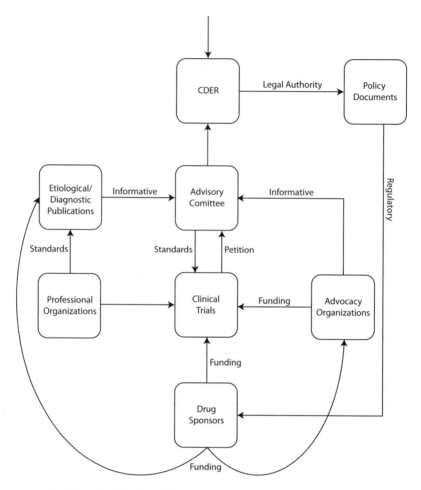

FIGURE 6.4. Network of DACs and pharmaceutical approval, detailing the calibration of influences within the MIC that have contributed to the indication of Lyrica for the treatment of FMS. The combined efforts of diagnostics, radiology, and pathology have established the legitimacy of FMS within RCTs, a legitimacy sanctioned by the peer-review process. Furthermore, pharmaceuticals' desire to expand the Lyrica market contributed to the proliferation of FMS-favorable RCTs. The new glut of data when presented to the AAC ultimately resulted in the establishment of a new policy document: the Lyrica indication.

of the AAC meeting. Pfizer is the manufacturer of Lyrica, and Sanofi (Genzyme's parent company) unsuccessfully attempted to secure FDA approval for another FMS drug.

All in all, this presents a much more complicated network of articulations between the AAC and industry. (See fig. 6.4 for a full elaboration.)

Pharmaceutical corporations fund the trials on which AAC decisions are based. They fund the research of several AAC participants. They fund a large part of the NFA and therefore, potentially, a portion of the patient representative's salary. Indeed, as figure 6.4 suggests, industry has the longest and most densely articulated enrollments of any other entity involved in regulating drug approval for FMS. Likely, this is the case for other drugs and diseases as well.

The AAC meeting was conducted from 8:05 a.m. to 2:54 p.m., with a forty-minute lunch recess. The meeting centered around six formal presentations, subsequent question-and-answer periods, and a final committee discussion. The formal presentations, synthetic recitations of then cutting-edge research on FMS etiology, diagnosis, and possibilities for pharmacologic treatment, included (1) Historical Background on Fibromyalgia, (2) Basic Mechanisms, (3) Post-ACR Diagnostic Criteria, (4) A Patient's Perspective, (5) Outcomes: Multi-System Impact, and (6) Charge to the Committee. A space on the program was designated for public comment, but no members of the public signed up for the opportunity.[1] As noted above, the primary and stated purpose of the meeting was to develop drug efficacy claim language that would include FMS. In his opening remarks, FDA staff member Dr. James Witter outlined these goals:

> We have an interesting day, I think, set up. This has a potential to be an historic day. We're going to be discussing something today that we have not at this point really discussed in any great detail at an advisory committee meeting, and we have a task today, which is essentially to go about and have a discussion about creating a claim for fibromyalgia. (Food and Drug Administration, 2003, p. 11)

Although these opening remarks identified several subsidiary goals including informational presentations (essentially a document of the state of science on FMS), the thrust of Dr. Witter's remarks indicated the primacy of the claim and label development goals. His further elaboration on the purpose and utility of claims language is instructive at this point:

> So we talk about claims and labels. Let's make sure that we are on the same page. It's stated quite often that although label claims have legal and regulatory uses, their central purpose is to inform health care providers and patients about the documented, and I stress documented, benefits and risks associated with a product. So claims, therefore, describe clinical benefits and that's really

what we're going to be trying to address today. What are those clinical benefits? The better that a product is labeled, the more effective it is then to allow for a useful risk management program which is something that we're all very much concerned about these days. (Food and Drug Administration, 2003, pp. 12–13)

Despite this focus on the development of claims and labeling as the primary issue at hand, the bulk of the debate was less focused.

The meeting transcript (Food and Drug Administration, 2003) provides contradictory information about the makeup of this group of interlocutors. I do not mean to say that there was any disagreement about who was in attendance. What is less clear is the perspectives and opinions that committee members brought to the debate. Toward the end of the meeting, FDA staff member Dr. Lee Simon reflected on his efforts to assemble the committee: "We tried to construct a committee that was part skeptic, part expert, part experience, and I think we really achieved that. Some people came totally disbelieving there was any reason to have this discussion" (Food and Drug Administration, 2003a, p. 252). Despite this claim to inclusivity and skepticism, I was unable to locate any discourse in the transcripts that indicated a strong objection to an FMS-based claim. Indeed, Dr. Clauw reinforces this notion with his tongue-in-cheek hedge about some data presented on one of his presentation slides: "Now, for any of the fibromyalgia skeptics that might be hiding in the room here, I'm not going to leave this slide up very long because this slide by itself will lead people to think that fibromyalgia isn't really real" (Food and Drug Administration, 2003a, p. 116). Such contradictory information makes it quite difficult to determine the true level of skepticism in the room, or if, in fact, the meeting was largely procedural.

Nevertheless, it is clear that at the time of this meeting those advocating for the development of claims and labels for FMS were still presumed to have the burden of proof regarding the ontological status of the disease itself. Indeed, in the 253-page transcript, 141 pages are devoted to documenting the reality of FMS. Much of this discourse takes the same form as the arguments for FMS that can be found in chapter 4. Speakers deployed the PR / WT accounts of etiological, diagnostic, and neuroimaging research and on FMS, all while calibrating each of the areas of research practice to one another. Additionally, the patient representative provided personal testimony and survey data on the experiential reality of FMS. Once again, CBD through neuroimaging data was a recurrent feature of the FMS ontologization discourse. fMRI data was provided both to address etiological concerns and to reinforce the possibility of diagnostic differentiation. PowerPoint slides accompanying the presentation showed over a dozen representative neuroimages and several additional data displays of fMRI data.

The transcript's remaining 112 pages of presentation and discussion are devoted to discussing the range of acceptable clinical trial designs for testing any potential FMS drugs. Specifically, these discussions centered on (1) what would be measured (pain, quality of life, and so on), (2) the length of the trial (three versus six months), (3) what efforts to manage comorbid conditions should be included, and (4) the ethics of placebo design. In clinical trial research for pain conditions, it is often considered unethical to deploy a true placebo-controlled study. Doing so would result in a study group that was untreated for pain, something generally considered a violation of clinical ethics. A typical alternative is a study design that includes "analgesic rescue"—that is, the availability of alternative pain killers so the placebo group (or the treatment group should the drug prove ineffective) does not have to suffer. As previously mentioned, no vote was taken. Nevertheless, the tone at the end of the meeting does represent the emergence of a consensus. The general tenor of the closing conversation suggests agreement about (1) the need for an approved FMS treatment, (2) the importance of treatment evaluation by the most robust RCT possible, and (3) a list of possible measures of drug efficacy. As previously mentioned, this consensus formed the foundation for Pfizer's request to add FMS to the list of indications for Lyrica. The summary review documentation notes, on numerous occasions, the use of a modified version of the AAC recommendations as the foundation for review.

In documenting this foundation for the establishment of the first drug approved by the FDA for FMS, I have nearly finished tracing the dense entanglements that can be activated in the approval process. However, the case of FMS and Lyrica can be traced even further, and here again is another potential entrée for pharmaceutical funding as a mode of network activation. FMS's long status as a contested illness and deep dissatisfaction due to lack of legitimacy and treatment options have paved the way for the establishment of a number of different advocacy organizations like the NFA. The Fibromyalgia Network, the National Fibromyalgia and Chronic Pain Association, Advocates for Fibromyalgia, Treatment, Education, and Research, the National Fibromyalgia Research Association, and the American Fibromyalgia Syndrome Association are a few such organizations. Their members participate in a wide variety of activities including research funding, community outreach, patient support groups, and lobbying efforts. It is these lobbying efforts that are of particular relevance here. Many of these organizations have coordinated congressional letter-writing campaigns that have resulted in opportunities for members of the FMS clinical and patient communities to testify before Congress. Indeed, the Fibromyalgia Network credits "congressional pressure" with increasing the availability of NIH funding for FMS research (Fibromyalgia Network, n.d.). And the AAC meeting explicitly acknowledged that joint workshops with the NIH paved the way for their work developing a claim. All told, this provides us with an increasingly complex model of the MIC and the nodes activated during drug approval and disease legitimization. Figure 6.5 further elaborates figure 6.4 in accounting for the added complexity of advocacy, lobbying, and congressional pressure.

Once again, I wish very much that the analysis of this data set enabled me to provide a clear indication as to the success of the FDA in its rarefactive mission. It does indeed seem possible that, from time to time, the FDA inhibits the interests of Big Pharma and, in so doing, does its job on behalf of the people. Certainly, the removal of "associated with sinusitis" from the list of acceptable uses for OTC cold medicine is one such instance. It is equally possible that the FDA may, in the future, choose to disallow "sinus headache" as a brand name for OTC cold medicines. Additionally, I would point to other research I have conducted documenting the role of DACs in challenging the interests of pharmaceutical complies (Teston & Graham, 2012; Teston, Graham, Baldwinson, Li & Swift, 2014). These articles explore how the Oncologic Drugs Advisory Committee revoked the popular cancer drug Avastin's indication for breast cancer at great financial cost to big pharmaceuticals. Nevertheless, in spite of these hopeful signs, the length and strength of the pharmaceutical industry's network of articulation within and around the FDA suggests that these cases are the exception rather than the rule.

Despite these valid concerns, I'm hesitant to come down too hard on members of the FDA. While the shift from sinus headache to migraine and the legitimization of FMS have certainly paved the way for a tremendous amount of money to transfer from patients to industry, these moves also seem to have opened up new avenues of treatment for unserved and underserved patient populations. Member of the AAC may well have been aware of the economic consequences of legitimizing FMS. However, what was the alternative? To continue to tell millions of suffering individuals that their disorder was unrecognized and they should not seek treatment? Obviously, this is an untenable response. Similarly, if migraineurs are truly being misdiagnosed, then they too deserve proper

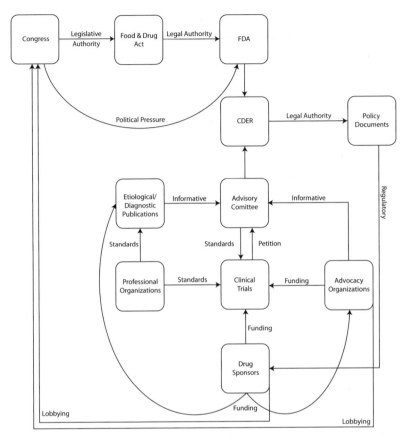

FIGURE 6.5. Lobbying activities and political pressure on pharmaceuticals approval. Elaborating figure 6.4, this diagram details the role of pharmaceutical funding and advocacy organization efforts to influence pharmaceutical regulation by enrolling legislative authority and political pressure in their programs of action.

treatment. Perhaps members of the OTC Cold and Cough Panel recognize the potential shift from OTC sinus headache medicine to triptans and are, therefore, hesitant to extend the revocation of the sinusitis indication to proprietary names enforcement.

Beyond the Hegemonic Fallacy

While I cannot end this chapter on a resoundingly hopeful note in the face of hegemonic claims about Big Pharma and the MIC, I think these cases, however aporia inducing, still demonstrate the failure of the hegemonic fallacy and the need to transcend two-world thinking in humanistic, critical, new materialist studies of medicine. If my analyses say only one thing about the MIC, it's that the networks of calibration surrounding the FDA are variable and subject to differential activation. The Food and Drug Act outlines a network of calibration and rarefaction that centers on the FDA (fig. 6.1). This model, however, shuffles immediately, activating some assemblages and deactivating others when the analysis zeros in on labeling claim rarefaction in the case of the sinus headache. As figure 6.2 demonstrates, certain network pathways are activated by this calibrating discourse that might not have been activated in other cases. Proprietary name rarefaction (fig. 6.3) activates the Divisions of Drug Labeling and Medical Error, which are not at play in the labeling claim revision. The labeling claim revision is played out in the *Federal Register* and only includes the AAAAI because they chose to comment on this issue. And in none of these cases was a DAC activated. The FMS claim construction hearing offered at the AAC activates an entirely different calibrating network (fig. 6.4). And the lobbying efforts of patient-advocacy organizations encouraged Congress to get involved with the FDA with an atypical level of detail (fig. 6.5).

The differential activations of the MIC points to failure of the hegemonic fallacy, which has no choice but to construe Big Pharma as all powerful and patients as naive and compliant subjects. While neither my investigation of the sinus headache nor of FMS offers a wholly hopeful vision of the FDA as effective rarefactive police, they both demonstrate that the monolithic model of Big Pharma is simply untenable. Although the full regulatory power of the FDA is seldom wholly utilized, the agency's location at the center of the MIC allows it to calibrate different regimes of practice so as to authorize certain ontologies and the diseases they stage. The clinical practices of neurology trump OTC self-medication and subsequently sinus headaches become migraines. The clinical practices of rheumatology when detoured (again through neurology) trump the practices of those who would dismiss fibromyalgics as mentally ill. And in each of these cases, the calibrating efforts at the center of the MIC have a profound impact on the practical regimes of engagement that stage the medical ontologies in question. What individual clinicians can and cannot do in their local sites of practice changes. Psychotherapy and Sudafed Sinus Headache give way to Lyrica and triptans, staging new ontologies that authorize FMS and reject the sinus headache.

Finding the Groove

In order to achieve optimum boat speed while sailing close-hauled (45 degrees off the wind for most sailboats), it is essential to find an ideal alignment between two competing pressure systems. The sail and the keel function as an airfoil and a hydrofoil, respectively, generating opposing lift vectors. When the two lift forces come into optimal balance, both in terms of intensity and vertical alignment, there is a noticeable acceleration. Sailors affectionately refer to this moment as "finding the groove." One artifact of the acceleration is that that boat seems to lower ever so slightly, as though there were some hidden track just below the ocean surface waiting for the keel to lock into place. Finding the groove is difficult. It requires an impressive combination of knowledge and dexterity to quickly and efficiently align the opposing pressure systems and "lock the keel into place." Finding the groove is a very subtle maneuver. Whether it is a twelve-foot dinghy or a fifty-foot yacht, the skipper must inch the boat carefully into place. When people have a great deal of difficulty finding the groove, it is typically a result of hypercorrection. The skipper recognizes that the boat is not in the groove and throws the tiller or wheel to one side, forcing the boat to quickly cut across the groove rather than settle into it. Hypercorrection after hypercorrection often results in a visible sinusoidal wake across the groove. Subsequently, skippers are trained to look backward and ask themselves, "Do I see a straight line or a snaking S curve into the distance?"

It is time to take a lesson from sailors. It is time to look backward and to see the oh-so-obvious S curve that indicates critical theorists, STS scholars, and rhetoricians have not found the groove. The moderns set an admittedly suboptimal course. However, the postmodern account of scientific knowledge represents an obvious hypercorrection against the positivist and materialist accounts of scientific discovery. The postmoderns, recognizing that the moderns were not quite on the right tack, threw the wheel hard over and cut straight across the groove, and very possibly into irons (dead upwind with no momentum). The anti-representationalist strain of object-oriented new materialism is also a hypercorrection against the postmodernism that came before it. Recognizing that the postmodern critique of modernism went too far in eliding the agency of the material, object-oriented new materialists threw the wheel hard over again. In so doing, they've come out of irons and started picking up a lot of speed, but they still have not found the groove. This is why I offer rhetorical-ontological inquiry as a viable alternative. It is an adjustment back to the center rather than a hypercorrection. It is a slow and deliberate tweaking of the wheel as part of a concerted effort not to undo what came before, but to find the groove and balance out the opposing pressure systems that demand either object-oriented or human-centered accounts.

Of course, I am not the first to recognize that a more modest course correction may be in order. In this respect *The Politics of Pain Medicine* constitutes something of a complement to Andrew Pickering's (1995) insights in *The Mangle of Practice*. Pickering, writing amid the postmodern hypercorrection, argued:

> Whenever [the sociology of scientific knowledge] detects a tendency for the action to be located elsewhere—a decentering of the human subject—it undertakes the police action already discussed. Any trace of nonhuman agency is immediately recuperated by translating it into an account of nonhuman agency that is attributed straight back to human subjects. . . . But the mangle, like the actor-network approach, corrodes the distinctions these discourses and disciplines enforce. It is not just that the mangle or the actor-network multiple sites of agency, trying to keep both human and nonhuman agency in view at the same time. Rather, in their somewhat different ways, the mangle and the actor-network insist on the constitutive intertwining and reciprocal interdefinition of human and material agency. (pp. 25–26)

Rejecting the postmodern police action, Pickering offers a compelling account of bubble chambers in particle physics to demonstrate that while, as social constructivists have argued, theories are made, they are not simply made up. Reality exerts a limiting influence so that not any theory can be made—and what theories *can* be made must constantly be refined in "the mangle of scientific practice" that coordinates the "dance of agency" between humans with their theories and nonhumans with their traces.

Like *The Mangle of Practice*, *The Politics of Pain Medicine* offers a more subtle course correction. It aims to help find the groove. However, unlike Pickering, I am responding not only to the postmodern hypercorrection but also to the more recent hypercorrection embodied by the object-oriented new materialist rejection of representation. To that end, as I close *The Politics of Pain Medicine*, I will offer a brief calibration of my own. In so doing, I start with some adding up, as Mol would put it—briefly revisiting the key moments in this book that point toward the necessity of a modest course correction in accounting for acts of representation. Then I will offer a short autopraxiography that explores future directions for rhetorical-ontological inquiry. And finally, I will close with a calibrating reflection on the overlapping insights of rhetorical-ontological inquiry and nonmodern approaches to pain.

Adding It Up

Certainly, the practices of clinical medicine do not occur in a vacuum. Indeed, health-care providers—be they physicians, nurses, chiropractors, or physical therapists—are subject to a "scope of practice" document that outlines what they can and cannot do. Any of these scopes of practice include scalpels, IV fluids, bacteria, clot matter, spinal cord stimulators, nociceptive impulses, neurotransmitters, and a whole host of other objects that are actively involved in the ontological performance. Nevertheless, discursive activity in the form of disciplinary tradition and federal regulations places clear limitations on clinical practice. Clinicians cannot do whatever they want, and they in turn cannot stage any ontology. However, as the practices of pain science and management indicate, individual clinicians can and do stage multiple pain ontologies including the semiotic, the biomechanical, and the empirical-discursive. And, indeed, the practices of pain management can and do stage emergent ontologies such as the nonmodern-practical with its biopsychosocial metaphysics and the nonmodern-discursive with its phenomenology of suffering.

Furthermore, this recognition tells us something important about Collen's pain cryptex from my introduction (fig. I.1). Ultimately, the cryptex expresses a (post-)modernist anxiety. It posits a real essential pain below the surface where coded and conflicting representations float. Rereading the cryptex through rhetorical-ontological inquiry and praxiography, in contrast, suggests that "solving" the cryptex is not so difficult. Unlike the cryptex of Brown's *Da Vinci Code*, there is not just one single sequence that unlocks the hidden chamber inside. Rather, many combinations open the cryptex. The manifold doings of multiple practical regimes of engagement "solve" the cryptex and reveal a pain. Note that: *a* pain. So the new challenge of the praxiographic cryptex is not unearthing *the* secret. Rather, the new challenge springs from the recognition that the process of solving the cryptex changes what is inside, revealing *a* secret. Each of the many solutions reveals (stages) a different pain. In fact, there is something of a productive resonance between the notion of the cryptex and the practices of calibration. Solving the cryptex exemplifies the deft and delicate maneuverings required to align the diverse practices and representations of pain science in order to reveal or stage a pain ontology and attendant disease metaphysics. Certainly, as the work of this book demonstrates, when fledgling or marginalized ontologies come on the scene, the practices of calibration are necessary to adjudicate the emergent or contested scopes of practice and metaphysics of disease. Subjective patient report, brain scans, laboratory findings, and clinical judgment are aligned around the circumference of the cryptex so as to open up new pain possibilities (in the case of FMS) or to forever lock away questionable pains (the sinus headache).

Taken in total, the collected cases of the MPG Journal Club, the disciplines of radiology, pathology, and diagnostics, and the networks of the MIC provide future rhetorical-ontological inquiry with a solid start toward developing a taxonomy of calibration practices and complementary rhetorical, technological, and authorizing institutional resources. My analyses of attempts to (1) foster a biopsychosocial approach to pain, (2) legitimize FMS, and (3) exorcise the sinus headache provide rhetorically oriented ontographers and new materialist rhetoricians with five modes of calibration, three types of authorizing resources, and three forms of discursive instantiation that may well provide insight into other spaces of calibration. The details of this calibration suite are available in table C.1.

While I think this suite provides an excellent foundation for continued rhetorical-ontological inquiry, I would be remiss if I did not outline some of the possible future horizons of inquiry that extend beyond calibrating practices but are equally appropriate to rhetorical-ontological inquiry. And this is where my autopraxiography really comes to the fore. Specifically, as I reflect on the future directions for rhetorical-ontological inquiry, I have identified two essential avenues for future work. First, rhetorical-ontological inquiry would benefit from increased attention to

TABLE C.I **Calibration suite identifying and defining the modes of calibration, authorizing resources, and discursive instantiations explored in *The Politics of Pain Medicine***

Modes of calibration	
Cross-ontological calibration	The practices of coordinating and aligning divergent ontologies so as to stage/highlight/celebrate multiplicity
Calibration by detour (CBD)	The practices of warranting/legitimizing a new or marginalized ontology by aligning it to the practices of an authoritative ontology
Constitutive calibration	The practices of coordinating or aligning divergent practical regimes of engagement so as to warrant/legitimize a particular ontology or object (disease) metaphysics
Rarefactive calibration	The practices of coordinating or aligning divergent practical regimes of engagement so as to exorcise/delegitimize a particular ontology or object metaphysics
Adding up	The practices of collecting and tabulating insights from multiple ontologies without attempting to coordinate, align, or reconcile differences

Authorizing resources	
Institutions of rarefaction	Organizations like academic disciplines, medical subspecialties, and federal regulatory agencies that are authorized or appointed specifically to perform rarefactive and constitutive calibration
Principles of rarefaction	Field/institution-specific, typically obscured material-semiotic assemblages that serve as obligatory passage points for rarefactive and/or constitutive calibration
Black-boxed technologies	Technologies whose legitimacy is so widely accepted in a given field that their inner workings are not subject to interrogation or criticism

Discursive instantiations	
Functional stasis	The process whereby foundational questions are raised, adjudicated, and resolved in calibration. The complexities of cross-ontological calibration typically require addressing nested stases whose resolution serves to buttress the resolution of prior stases
Trope shifting	The discursive component of black boxing whereby propositional metaphors shift into metonymy or synecdoche so as to more rapidly elide the complexities of a technology
Warranting topoi	Powerful commonplaces in a specific field or institutions that can be used to authorize lines of argument

the reciprocal relationships among words and things at sites of practical regimes of engagement. And second, it would benefit from the development of interventional forms of practice. Subsequently, I will close this book with a brief speculative exegesis envisioning what these new horizons of inquiry might look like and how rhetoricians and STS scholars could bring them into being.

Words and Things

Certainly, as my gloss of Pickering above suggests, I am not the first to argue for an increased focus on the reciprocal relationships among words and things at sites of practical activity. Indeed, the argument to do so has been a mainstay of actor-network theory (ANT) since its inception. Nowhere in the ANT oeuvre is this better exemplified than, perhaps, in Latour's (1999) analysis of soil researchers in *Pandora's Hope*. In the passage below, Latour describes the efforts of a soil scientist to properly categorize a bit of dirt using the Munsell color code:

> At this moment, the power of standardization . . . is less interesting to me than a stupefying technical trick—the little holes that have been pierced above the shades of color. Though seemingly always out of reach, the threshold between local and global can now be crossed instantaneously. Still, it takes some skill to insert the soil sample into the Munsell code. In order for the soil sample to qualify as a number, René must in fact be able to match, superpose, and align the local clod of earth, which he holds in his hand with the standardized color chosen as reference. To accomplish this, he passes the soil sample beneath the openings made in the notebook and, by successive approximations, selects the color closest to that of the sample. There is, as I have said, a complete rupture at each stage between the "thing" part of each object and its "sign" part, between the tail of the soil sample and its head. That abyss is all the wider because our brains are incapable of memorizing color with precision. Even if the soil sample and the standard were no farther apart than ten or fifteen centimeters, the width of the notebook, this would be enough for René's brain to forget the precise correspondence between the two. The only way the resemblance between a standardized color and a soil sample can be established is by piercing holes in the pages that allow us to align the rough surface of the lump of soil with the bright and uniform surface of the standard. With less than a millimeter of distance separating them, then and only then can they be read synoptically. Without the holes, there can be no alignment, no precision, no reading, and therefore no transmutation of local earth into universal code. Across the abyss of matter and form, René throws a bridge. It is a footbridge, a line, a grappling hook. (Latour, 1999, pp. 59–60)

Here Latour offers a praxiography before its time. He provides the reader with an account of the microscale local practices of soil scientists. However, he does not only focus on the objects, the soil, the plastic board.

ANT, like Pickering's mangle and my rhetorical-ontological inquiry, is a more modest course correction. It intentionally seeks to balance the opposing forces of human- and object-centered accounts. It works to find the groove. As Latour's praxiography indicates, the plastic board that supports the Munsell code is meaningless without that code. The soil scientist, in the langue of Mol and rhetorical-ontological inquiry, calibrates the soil sample to the code by detouring it though the wonderfully simple coding device. Words (codes) are calibrated to objects (soil) as an essential part of the practical regimes of engagement of pedology.

Examples of similar calibrations abound in the practices of pain science and medicine. The visual-analog scale (VAS) is a primary exemplar. Patients are called to perform two calibrating translations. They must imagine how the pain they feel would manifest on their face and calibrate that imaginary face to the smiley (or frowny) line drawings of the VAS. The calibrations of neuroimaging offer another primary example. The central nervous system dysregulation of FMS is made manifest for patient and clinician alike as blood flow is translated into radioactive scatter that is translated through algorithms and into images. The representational, whether mathematical or visual, is an essential part of the practices of neuroimaging. A praxiography of neuroimaging that only addressed oxygen, hemoglobin, radionucleotides, scintillating devices, silicone chips, and computer pixels would miss the essential contributions of the algorithm and the color scale.

Again, this is not an entirely novel insight. This is a course correction. I revisit the point here because I worry that my training as a rhetorician and my interests in the political dimensions of pain science and management has pulled my inquiry, necessarily, into the metapractical regimes of calibration. Furthermore, the hypercorrections of the aforementioned object-oriented strains of new materialism serve to reinforce this potential dichotomy in their total rejection of representation. As a result, I would hate for my readers to think that this speaks to the limits of rhetorical-ontological inquiry. To be sure, the networks of calibration surrounding local regimes of practice in any scientific or medical area are an ideal site for rhetorical-ontological inquiry. However, they are certainly not the only possible sites. So as I speculate, all too briefly, on the future possibilities for rhetorical-ontological inquiry, I would point to an emerging stream of new materialism as an ideal space for helping to extend rhetorical-ontological inquiry more fully into local sites of practice and therefore moderate necessary course corrections. This emerging trend comes from new materialism's reengagement with thing theory.

Heidegger's (1971) thing theory famously offers two primary modes of interfacing with objects/things/stuff. In so doing, he outlines a critical distinction between the thing (*Ding*) and the object (*Geganstand*). The German is essential here. Heidegger could have just as easily written about the *Objekt* and been well understood by his contemporaries. In choosing *Genganstand* (literally, that which stands against), he highlights the object's necessary participation in the orders of representation. *Das Ding*, on the other hand, precedes theory, existing in the orders of practice and doing. And here, it offers a great potential for synergistic entanglement with praxiography. Furthermore, much clarity is brought to the distinction between *Ding* and *Geganstand* in reading it against Heidegger's theory of tool-being. In *Being and Time* (2008), Heidegger distinguishes between *vorhanden* (present-to-hand) and *zuhanden* (ready-to-hand). In the famous example of the hammer, a perfectly functioning hammer articulated into the practice of carpentry is *zuhanden*. Its being recedes from notice, although it is still implicated in an order of activity, a regime of practice, that of carpentry. If the hammer were to break, however, it would become *vorhanden* and subject to theoretical attention of the carpenter, who must now assess and then fix or replace the hammer. For Heidegger, things are *zuhanden* and objects are *vorhanden*.

In other words, to be an object, to be *vorhanden*, is to stand against (*Gegenstand*) a subject in the order of representation. As Heidegger writes:

> An independent, self-supporting thing may become an object if we place it before us, whether in immediate perception or by bringing it to mind in a recollective re-presentation. However, the thingly character of the thing does not consist in its being a represented object, nor can it be defined in any way in terms of the objectness, the over-againstness, of the object. (1971, p. 167)

As mentioned above, several emergent strains of new materialism embrace thing theory and tool-being directly. Latour (2004), for example, uses the thing/object distinction to reinforce his proposed division between "matters of fact" and "matters of concern." In so doing, he argues that we need to take more seriously the thingyness of objects—that is, the ways that objects circulate within and are constituted by practical (including discursive) activity.

Another powerful example comes from Thomas Rickert's (2013) *Ambient Rhetoric*. The foreword to this book prefaces his use of Heidegger in shifting the reader's attention from *vorhanden* to *zuhanden*:

The project suggests we take as provisional starting points the dissolution of the subject-object relation, the abandonment of representationalist theories of language, an appreciation of nonlinear dynamics and the process of engagement, and the incorporation of the material word as integral to human action and interaction, including rhetorical arts. . . . World in this sense is not just the material environs, that is, the "mundane" bedrock of reality, but also the involvements and cares that emerge within and alongside the material environment and that in turn work to bring presence to the environs in the mode that they currently take. World, then, is simultaneously *immanent and transcendent* to each agent—and that includes nonhuman elements. (Rickert, 2013, xii–xiii, emphasis added)

As both Rickert and Latour suggest, Heidegger's thing is not solely defined in opposition to *Geganstand*, but also, in its own right, through the play of gathering and doing. Heidegger (1971) takes the question of *das Ding* to task through a diligent exploration of a typical philosophical desk object, a water jug. Heidegger's jug is not an object of our theoretical attention, but a thing that does stuff. It *holds* water, for one. It actively keeps the liquid from spilling out on the table. The jug *takes in* water. It *keeps* water. It *pours* water. For Heidegger, the jug's being is all of these doings and potential doings simultaneously. To this account of doing, Heidegger also adds *gathering*:

Neither the general, long outworn meaning of the term "thing," as used in philosophy, or the Old High German meaning of the word thing, however, are of the least help to us in our pressing need to discover and give adequate thought to the essential source of what we are now saying about the nature of the jug. However, one semantic factor in the old usage of the world thing, namely "gathering," does speak to the nature of the jug as we earlier had it in mind. The jug is a thing neither in the sense of the Roman *res*, nor in the sense of the medieval *ens*, let alone in the modern sense of object. The jug is a thing insofar as it things. (1971, p. 177)

In typical maddening Heideggerian fashion, a thing is a thing insofar as it things thingly. That is, the ontology of things lies at the intersections of doing, gathering, and presence. A thing is not forever locked in the order of representation, but it is rather a coparticipant in the doing of gatherings. As such, thing (as opposed to object) provides a ready-made term for addressing the recalcitrance of being and the ontologies staged

by practical regimes of engagement without the doomed attempt of trying to separate *Geganstand* from that which it stands against, as the anti-
representational object-oriented new materialist would have it.

So what is the benefit for the future of rhetorical-ontological inquiry?
A more modest course correction is made possible. Under the rubric of
thing theory—the coherence of doing, gathering, and presence—one
need neither elide representation nor perform the social constructivist police action identified by Pickering. Things thing thingly. And if in
their gathering and doing, they gather through blood flow and radioactive decay, that gathering is not ontologically distinct from their gathering
through algorithms and images. Put another way, thing theory allows us
to move past the two-world problem and its never-ending recapitulation
of (as Foucault put it and Rickert acknowledges) the question of *les mots
et choses*, of words and things. Through thing theory, future rhetorical-
ontological inquiry might transform the problem into a dictum, *les mots
sont choses*: words are things. And thus we have a viable approach for an
integrated form of inquiry that can go all the way from the microscale, local practices of smashing soil through a hole on a color chart or a patient
selecting a representative smiley/frowny face all the way up to the networks of calibration of the Environmental Protection Agency, in the first
case, or the MIC, in the second.

Interventional Praxiography

As I continue this autopraxiography, it is now time to ask potentially
uncomfortable questions about what ontology is staged by rhetorical-
ontological inquiry. The answer, I'm afraid, is that it is rather clearly
empirical-discursive. Indeed, praxiography might well be the neuroimaging of rhetoric and STS. It involves an iterative series of ocular and inscriptive practices so as to create an account of doings. Recognizing this
tension, Mol's final chapter offers a not-uncompelling defense of praxiography as a form of interventional doing. She argues, somewhat persuasively, that "methods are not a way of opening a window on the world,
but a way of interfering with it. They act, they *mediate* between an object
and its representations. One way or another. Inevitably" (2002, p. 155).
However, Mol is ultimately more comfortable with this defense of praxiography than I am. It is perhaps easier for her, given the relative newness of empirical research methods in philosophy (Mol, 2002; Ashcroft,

2003; Holm & Jonas, 2004; Ives, 2008; Ives & Draper, 2009), to understand praxiography as a radically new form of doing. Indeed, it is quite strikingly different when compared to Heidegger's rumination on the nearest object at hand. Nevertheless, praxiography clearly owes a lot to ethnography, as Mol (2002) readily admits (p. 7). And it is equally clear from the self-reflective discourse of the ethnomethodologist that ethnography is a practice of looking.

Indeed, Clifford Geertz's (1973) famous account of ethnography highlights both the practices of looking and the importance of looking at words:

> To *look* at the symbolic dimensions of social action—art, religion, ideology, science, law, morality, commonsense—is not to turn away from the existential dilemmas of life for some empyrean realm of emotionalized forms; it is to plunge into the midst of them. The essential vocation of the interpretive anthropology is not to answer our deepest questions, but to make available to us answers that others, guarding other sheep in other valleys, have given, and thus to include them in the *consultable record of what man has said*. (p. 30, emphasis added)

Glossing Geertz, rhetorical ethnographer Carl Herndl (1991) offers a sort of autopraxiography of ethnography. In so doing, he crafts a compelling account of the central role of inscriptive practices as a necessary analogy to observing (looking) in the doings of ethnography:

> Clifford Geertz points out, "the ethnographer 'inscribes' social discourse, he writes it down. In so doing he turns it from a passing event, which exists only in its own moment of occurrence, into an account, which exists in its inscription and can be reconsulted" (19). The result is that the "data" to which we return to write ethnography is not an experience but the already textual representation of fieldnotes. Furthermore, constructing the ethnographic account is a rhetorical activity. "We measure the cogency of our explications," Geertz argues, "not against a body of uninterpreted data . . . but against the power of the scientific imagination to bring us into touch with the lives of strangers" (16). As readers we judge ethnography by the way it makes the strange or alien seem familiar and palpably real. The imaginative power which wins readers' assent is a matter not simply of knowledge but also of rhetorical skill. Ethnographies persuade readers not by the power of factual description but by employing the narrative structures, textual tropes, and argumentative topoi developed by the ethnographic genre. Geertz's own notion of "thick description" is a case in point. It

is a highly stylized form of verisimilitude that has become a standard in discussions of ethnographic method and functions as a textual strategy authorizing
attempts at ethnographic realism. (Herndl, 1991, p. 321)

Ultimately, I think an honest autopraxiography must recognize that the
lookings and inscriptions of praxiographic practice stage an empirical-
discursive ontology, just like neuroimaging. And it may even run the risk of
imperialist epistemic violence. Indeed, does my account of how neuroimperialism silences fibromyalgics in an attempt to speak for them offer any
more voice to those same fibromyalgics? I still purport to speak for them.

While it is essential to recognize the limits of empirical-discursive
praxiography, I do not argue that it should be thrown out of our repertoire of practices. In fact, this would be practically quite difficult given
the calibrating networks of the academy. Disciplines, peer review boards,
and promotion and tenure committees are all institutions of rarefaction
charged with policing the discourse of scholarship. In each of these institutions of rarefaction, a preference for empirical-discursive ontology
is notable. Certainly, every academic knows the story of at least one colleague who found her- or himself confronted by the need to calibrate her
or his avant-garde, artistic, or interventional scholarship to the fairly narrow principles of rarefaction deployed by tenure committees.

And beyond this pragmatic argument, I would argue that any area of
inquiry benefits from multiplicity. *The Politics of Pain Medicine* documents how the multiplicity of pain is staged by the multiplicity of practical regimes of engagement. Certainly, multiple pain practices stage an
empirical-discursive ontology, but the mere existence of this ontology is
not a detriment to pain. Rather, problems arise when calibrating efforts
attempt to remove all other ontologies from pain practice. The multiplicity of pain practices is what makes the biopsychosocial metaphysics of pain
possible. If all pain scientists and all pain managers did the same thing, an
invariably more limited pain ontology would be the only one available,
at great cost for patients. Furthermore, practical regimes of engagement
(such as neuroimaging) that stage an empirical-discursive ontology serve
as valuable resources for marginalized ontologies as they seek legitimacy.
While this is not unproblematic, I have to wonder if FMS would be so
widely accepted today if it were not for neuroimaging technologies. Ultimately, my analysis of pain points to the value and importance of a great
variety of practices in any area of inquiry. The rhetorical-ontological
inquiry presented in *The Politics of Pain Medicine* offers one suite of

practices—those that focus on interrogating the practices of calibration across a variety of networked institutions of rarefaction. My suggestion above that rhetorical-ontological inquiry might benefit from a detour through thing theory has the potential to authorize another set of practices that focus on interrogating the local practices of scientific inquiry in such a way that there is no ontological distinction between words and things. And finally, as rhetorical-ontological inquiry moves forward, it would further benefit from developing a more fully interventional form of inquiry.

In both critical and practical ways, rhetorical-ontological inquiry has the opportunity to contribute to either what Collins and Evans (2002) dub "working upstream" (p. 240) or what Haraway (1997) identifies as the "high-stakes game" of "shaping technoscience" (p. 50). Rhetorical-ontological inquiry can use its investigational resources to catalyze and assist interventional and emancipatory projects in a wide variety of domains. The calibration suite in table C.1 clearly demonstrates this possibility. If those practicing rhetorical-ontological inquiry ally themselves with those pursing social goods, the calibration suite provides a ready-made heuristic for analyzing the institutions of rarefaction, principles of rarefaction, and calibrating moves on which and with which positive change can be engineered. The development of interventional forms of praxiography, like the move toward interrogated local spaces of word/thing reciprocity, need not be built from the ground up. Like Latour's (2004) and Rickert's (2013) deployment of thing theory, many are already working with interventional methodologies that might be calibrated to the practices of rhetorical-ontological inquiry.

Primary among such efforts is the critical action research (CAR) of Blythe, Grabill, and Riley (2008). CAR, as the name suggests, is an outgrowth of long-standing efforts in participatory action research (PAR). PAR and CAR are both interventional in nature, but not quite in the same way. In an earlier work that points toward the establishment of CAR, Grabill (2006) argues that a systemic understanding of institutional spaces is necessary to understand the possibilities for positive change and contribute to interventional research goals:

> Contemporary institutions are the scene of struggle.... [T]he problem of agency is the problem of acting within systems of decision-making marked by organizational, epistemological, and discursive complexity. These institutional systems thoroughly penetrate our lives. (p. 159)

Building on this insight, Blythe, Grabill, and Riley (2008) argue for CAR, which is essentially a fusion of PAR and applied rhetoric. In some ways, it is a form of technical communications consulting. Ultimately, however, it is a nuanced research form with a constant attention to ethical outcomes. As the authors explain, CAR differs from PAR in that the ethnographers "conduct research on behalf of citizens rather than with them" (p. 7). Furthermore, in distancing itself from PAR and focusing on the articulations of groups and institutions, CAR productively sidesteps the hegemonic fallacy that can be so pervasive in postmodern interventional research. Blythe, Grabill, and Riley explore CAR through their work helping citizen-activists develop and refine their communications practices in the face of a proposed dredging project (with massive potential environmental consequence). In so doing, CAR helped the authors to develop a "map" that describes the community as "an articulation of groups of people and institutions, arrayed in relation to each other with respect to the dredging project" (p. 19). With a better understanding of the articulations in what I would call the networks of calibration surrounding the proposed dredging project, citizen-activists were more prepared to participate in the calibrating activities of that network.

Clearly, very similar work could be done with marginalized disease communities or to combat disturbing pharmaceutical initiatives. CAR-style mapping efforts could be combined with thing theory insights to map the networks of calibration that include humans and nonhumans, things and words. These mapping practices could then be iteratively combined with rhetorical-ontological insights into the principles of rarefaction and modes of calibration at work in the network in question. Thus, the suite of practices available for rhetorical-ontological inquiry can be productively extended and new ontologies that transcend the empirical-discursive might be staged. And as the available repertoire of rhetorical-ontological practice and ontologies proliferate, then rhetorically oriented ontographers and ontologically oriented STS scholars may well find themselves in the same position as the MPG—that is, with a manifest exigency to found their own space of calibration and collaboration.

Final Calibrations

While certainly there are many viable future horizons of inquiry within a rhetorical-ontological idiom, I do not want to overlook the insights that come from calibrating my initial efforts with the insights of the biopsychosocial. *The Politics of Pain Medicine* offers another contribution to the mounting pile of evidence demonstrating that the tired performances of the two-world hypothesis no longer play so well in the ontological theater. The practices required of contemporary rhetorical-ontological inquiry and pain science and medicine can no longer so easily stage the dominant ontologies of modernism and postmodernism. Whether it is new materialist academics or biopsychosocial pain specialists, the old scripts are not working anymore. The modernist distinction between objective clinical findings and subjective patient report fails to ethically serve patients with complex multicausal and/or marginalized diseases. The disease/illness dichotomy so popular in critical/cultural studies of medicine, it turns out, reinforces the line of demarcation between patient and physician, further enfranchising the singular "reality" of the disease over the manifold "perceptions" of the illness. Subsequently, the analytic move that recognizes the myth of two pains is turned back on itself, revealing such insights as pluralistic and therefore perspectival. That is, the two pains are not one pain, but rather many pains, multiple pains. Indeed, with the myth of two pains read against the clinical distinctions between nociceptive and psychogenic pain, we are forced to reimagine new horizons of inquiry focused on the biopsychosocial or even a phenomenology of suffering. While pain management clinicians recognize the manifest failure of the isolation of subspecialties to treat the complexities of nonmodern pain, rhetoricians and STS scholars must confront the kindred failure of the incommensurability thesis to explain what happens at disciplinary boundaries. Furthermore, in the broader networks of disease calibration, it is no longer so easy to accept the totalizing account of a Big Pharma run amok, nor to construe the marginalized patient advocacy group (with its pharmaceutical industry funding) as simply speaking truth to power.

The two-world problem and its correlative epistemic and hegemonic fallacies that underwrite these failed scripts has proven untenable for either rhetorical-ontological inquiry or pain science and medicine. But as it turns out, rejecting the two-world hypothesis is no easy task. Certainly, the postmodernists have been claiming to do so for years without actually accomplishing that aim. Additionally, the anti-representationalism of object-oriented new materialisms serves to tacitly reinforce this word/thing dichotomy as it authorizes a vision of hyper-incommensurability. Similarly, detours through neuroimaging enact a form of neuroimperialism where, in a clear act of epistemic violence, the marginalized are silenced through the re-presentation. Even when it comes to more

Notes

Introduction

1. While those less familiar with the work of Latour might read the rejection of the mind/body dichotomy as a postmodern (as opposed to nonmodern) move, I follow Latour's rejection of postmodernity as a mode of inquiry that inadvertently extends and reverses modernist binaries. I will revisit this argument in greater detail toward the end of this introduction.

2. From 2006 to 2008, I worked as a participant-observer with the MPG. Subsequently, the research into the MPG is firsthand, subject to human-subjects research oversight, and has been, therefore, pseudonymized. Both the organizational name of the MPG and the names of individual members are inventions. The pseudonyms presented in *The Politics of Pain Medicine* are consistent with my previous work exploring the MPG (Graham, 2009, 2011; Graham & Herndl, 2011, 2013). Since my exploration of the AAPM and the IASP has been based entirely on public discourse (with few exceptions that will be identified and pseudonymized), these organizational and individual names are accurate.

3. It is typical to provide quotations from ethnographic interviews using the citation practices of the style guide in use. In this case, APA requires a date to be provided within each in-text citation. However, I must decline to do so. In a study such as this, the primary risk to subjects is breach of confidentiality. The more accurate information I provide about each interview, the realization of that primary risk is increased, however slightly. I could provide fictitious dates to go with the pseudonyms, but given that interview transcripts cannot be ethically provided, it seems an unnecessary to contribute to the false "documentary power" (Herndl, 1991, p. 362) of ethnographic citations.

4. The list of scholarship on visual rhetoric is far too extensive to cite in detail. For starters, one might turn to Carolyn Handa's *Visual Rhetoric in a Digital World: A Critical Sourcebook* (2004) or Charles Kostelnick's *Shaping Information: The Rhetoric of Visual Conventions* (2003).

5. Rhetorical studies in the United States exists in multiple departmental locales, each with slightly different—though related—scholarly traditions. The
majority of rhetoric programs can be found in departments of English and departments of speech or communication studies. The programs in English departments
tended to arise out of an investment in teaching effective argumentation to first-
year students and technical communicators—though the tradition has extended
well beyond its pedagogical origin. Rhetoric in speech or communication studies departments generally hosts public speaking courses and has a long history of
scholarship in political oratory.

Chapter One

1. The IASP definition of pain will be discussed in greater detail in chapter 2.

2. The "modern synthesis" refers to the establishment of contemporary biology
that arose from the unification of evolutional science, genetics, ecology, cytology,
and other formerly independent areas of inquiry.

3. For convenience, I will refer to Hippocrates as the author of the Hippocratic
corpus.

4. The rise of statistics constitutes a profoundly powerful moment in the history
of science and medicine and will make an appearance in multiple ontologies. Although it arguably warrants its own section in this chapter, to do so would violate
my ethical commitment to the phylogenic model. This is a history of clades, and as
such the clade must be the organizing structure.

5. The methodological edicts that compose Foucault's analysis of the modern
episteme testify to his status as one progenitor of new materialism. The scientific
practices of modernity are staged front and center in his discussion of the new episteme. And while Foucault may have, at times, described the theory as a priori to
the practice, his focus on the material conditions of epistemic transformations pre-
figures the material-semiotic/ontological-epistemological collocations of multiple-
ontologies theory.

6. By broadly questioned, I refer to discourses outside of pain science proper.
Discussions of the ethics of research and animal rights are largely absent from general treatments of pain research, but Fishman and Berger (2000) provided readers
with a remarkably evenhanded discussion of the issue (pp. 83–84).

7. Though this chapter is largely a history of American medical discourse, this
period of French medicine is highly relevant. Even into the early twentieth century, the American medical community considered French medicine to be of the
highest quality. In fact, it was quite the fashion among well-to-do American physicians of the time to spend a year or two studying medicine in France after completing American medical school.

8. Both the WHO document and the 1965 FDA revision specifically reference
thalidomide.

Chapter Two

1. Members of the IASP and the MPG are active participants in the modernist discourses of biomedical research. As such, they would not describe their own efforts using the language of multiple ontologies. Rather, deploying a tacit version of the incommensurability thesis, they speak of the necessity of overcoming disciplinary silos in order to foster multidisciplinary care. As a result, I'll use the language of disciplines when representing the perspectives of MPG members and the language of multiple ontologies when conducting my analysis. To be sure, disciplines and ontologies are not the same thing, but neither are they unrelated. The academic metadiscourse that emerges from a coordinated suite of ontologies that, when it is self-policing, becomes a discipline.

2. A "board certification" is a recognition of expertise granted to health care providers by various professional organizations such as the American Board of Internal Medicine. Certification requires significant postgraduate education, and in some cases additional examination.

3. The MPG as described in this chapter is an accurate portrayal during the time of my participant observations. I have since learned that new regulations for pharmaceutical funding have resulted in a significant reduction in available funds and a subsequent reduction in attendance, forcing even MPG members to question the viability of the organization.

4. Though this genre could easily be identified as a variant of an article presentation or as an altogether different genre, I include it under the rubric of practice reflection because of the response it generates. The social conventions associated with each presentation genre differed in terms of the type of conversation and nature of discussion. Discussion conventions following both types of practice reflections could be the same and yet different from the other genres.

Chapter Three

1. During a member-checking presentation to the MPG, I was explaining how several of the members interviewed used the terminology of "conversion" to explain their motivations for joining the MPG. The audience members objected to the "religious overtones" of "conversion" and suggested that "epiphany" would be a better description.

Chapter Four

1. While it may seem indelicate to refer to members of patient populations by their diseases status, I do so in these cases so as to be faithful to my informants. Providers and patients alike, in each of these communities, routinely refer

to "migraineurs" and "fibromyalgics." In the case of FMS, this is even more important as a significant identity community has formed around the condition.

Chapter Five

1. Certainly, I am not the only scholar to identify this twin potential in Foucault.
New materialist Grosz (2010) highlights Foucault's genealogical work for its ability
to leverage the freedom from/freedom to dialectic (p. 141). She argues that feminist scholarship often focuses on freedom from concerns in regard to the repressive hypothesis and the escape from patriarchy. For Grosz, a primary affordance of
new materialism is its ability to shift the discourse of "freedom from" to "freedom
to" and its focus on horizons of possibility.

2. And this, too, is an area where Foucault's theory of discourse overlaps with
rhetorical stasis theory. The authority to speak and be recognized is a jurisdictional
issue in its own right—especially in the densely articulated networks of medical
science and clinical practice. When multiple powerful institutions vie to regulate
the same discourse, and authorize or prevent speakers from participating in that
discourse, jurisdiction becomes a key point of contention. Though my analysis in
this chapter will focus primarily on principles of rarefaction, the discourse of the
sinus headache is equally amenable to stasis analysis.

3. In this case, "external" does not mean nondiscursive. The external principles
of rarefaction are essentially the foundations of discourse. They are ontologically a
priori. In contrast, the "internal" principles arise within specific discourse and are
operationalized in different ways depending on their instantiation.

4. I take Foucault's "within the true" as an effective description of the metaphysics and epistemologies that arise from empirical-discursive ontologies. As he
explained in "The Discourse," the combined effects of the will-to-truth and the
will-to-knowledge "sketched out a schema of possible, observable, measurable
and classifiable objects"—that is, a collection of objects that can be recognized
(through discourse) as being, as existing.

5. Here I do not mean to commit the common and inappropriate conflation of
claim-warrant-data and the classical syllogism as appropriately pilloried by Keith
and Beard (2008). Rather, I merely aim to point to two overlapping lexicons for
the function of powerful argumentative structures. Neither sufficiently explains
the authorizing power of principles of rarefaction, but together they clarify the
boundaries of this essential element of rarefactive and constitutive calibration.

6. I surveyed approximately a dozen pathology textbooks located at two Iowa
medical schools (one osteopathic, one allopathic) and two medical archives. Their
publication dates range from the 1880s to 2008. At each of the medical schools,
I located the textbooks currently being used in the basic pathology courses for
medical students.

7. It should not go without noting that the medical testing industry is an economic powerhouse akin to the pharmaceutical industry. Testing representatives aggressively market and sell their tests to clinicians in much the same way as drug reps. Testing companies have even sponsored meetings of the MPG and provided speakers offering their products.

Chapter Six

1. Given the extremely well-organized (and largely well-funded) nature of FMS advocacy organizations, I must wonder how well publicized the special meeting was or how much time members of the public were given to respond to recruitment. Indeed, the patient representative noted during the meeting that she was appointed to the committee just "a couple of weeks" before the meeting date (FDA, 2003, p. 131).

References

Aho, K. (2008). Medicalizing mental health: A phenomenological alternative. *Journal of Medical Humanities, 29*, 243–259.

Althusser, L. (1971). *Lenin and philosophy and other essays by Louis Althusser*. New York: Monthly Review Press. (Original work published 1964–1969)

Ambrose, J. (1973). Computerized transverse axial scanning (tomography): Part II. Clinical application. *British Journal of Radiology, 46*, 1023–1047.

Amir, I., Yeo, J. C., & Ram, B. (2012). Audit of CT scanning of paranasal sinuses in patients referred with facial pain. *Rhinology, 50*(4), 442–446.

Anderson, J. M. (1996). Empowering patients: Issues and strategies. *Social Science and Medicine, 43*(5), 697–705.

Angell, M. (2005). *The truth about the drug companies: How they deceive us and what to do about it*. New York: Random House.

Annas, G. J. (2009). Globalized clinical trials and informed consent. *New England Journal of Medicine, 360*(20), 2050–2053.

Aristotle (2004). *On rhetoric*. (W. R. Roberts, Trans.). Mineola, NY: Dover Publications.

Arnold, L. M. (2006). New therapies in fibromyalgia. *Arthritis Research and Therapy, 8*, 212–232.

Ashcroft, R. E. (2003). Constructing empirical bioethics: Foucauldian reflections on the empirical turn in bioethics research. *Health Care Analysis, 11*(1), 3–13.

Atwood, M. (2003). *Oryx and crake*. New York: Anchor Books.

Bacon, F. (2000). Novum organon. In F. E. Baird & W. Kaufmann (Eds.), *Modern philosophy* (pp. 3–10). Englewood Cliffs, NJ: Prentice Hall.

Barclay, A. W. (1862). *A manual of medical diagnosis: Being an analysis of the signs and symptoms of disease*. Philadelphia: Blanchard and Lea.

Barker, K. K. (2011). Listening to Lyrica: Contested illnesses and pharmaceutical determinism. *Social Science & Medicine, 73*(6), 833–842.

Bazerman, C., & De Los Santos, R. A. (2005). Measuring incommensurability: Are toxicology and ecotoxicology blind to what the other sees? In R. A. Harris

(Ed.), *Rhetoric and incommensurability* (pp. 424–463). West Lafayette, IN: Parlor Press.

Bendelow, G. A., & Williams, S. J. (1995). Transcending the dualisms: Toward a sociology of pain. *Sociology of Health and Illness, 17*(2), 139–165.

Bennett, J. (2010a). A vitalist stop on the way to a new materialism. In D. Coole & S. Frost (Eds.), *New materialisms: Ontology, agency, and politics* (pp. 47–69). Durham, NC: Duke University Press.

Bennett, J. (2010b). *Vibrant matter: A political ecology of things.* Durham, NC: Duke University Press.

Bermingham, E. J. (1882). *An encyclopædic index of medicine and surgery.* New York: Bermingham & Co.

Blythe, S., Grabill, J. T., & Riley, K. (2008). Action research and wicked environmental problems: Exploring appropriate roles for researchers in professional communication. *Journal of Business and Technical Communication, 22,* 272–298.

Bogost, I. (2012). *Alien phenomenology, or What it's like to be a thing.* Minneapolis: University of Minnesota Press.

Bourdieu, P. (1988). *Homo academicus.* Palo Alto: Stanford University Press.

Braidott, R. (2002). *Metamorphoses: Towards a feminist theory of becoming.* Cambridge: Polity Press.

Braidotti, R. (2010). The politics of "life itself" and new ways of dying. In D. Coole and S. Frost (Eds.), *New materialisms: Ontology, agency, and politics* (pp. 201–220). Durham, NC: Duke University Press.

Brody, J. E. (2000, August 1). Fibromyalgia: Real illness, real answers. *New York Times,* p. 8F.

Brown, D. (2003). *The Da Vinci code.* New York: Doubleday.

Brown, T., & Murphy, E. (2010). Through a scanner darkly: Functional neuroimaging as evidence of a criminal defendant's past mental states. *Stanford Law Review, 62*(4), 1119–1208.

Bryant, L. (2011). *The democracy of objects.* Ann Arbor: Open Humanities Press.

Bunge, M. (2010). *Matter and mind: A philosophical inquiry.* New York: Springer.

Burke, K. (1969). *A Rhetoric of motives.* Berkeley: University of California Press.

Burton, S. (1996). Bakhtin, temporality, and modern narrative: Writing "the whole triumphant murderous unstoppable chute." *Comparative Literature, 48*(1), 39–64.

Cady, R. K., Dodick, D. W., Levine, H. L., Schreiber, C. P., Eross, E. J., Setzen, M., Blumenthal, H. J., Lumry, W. R., Berman, G. D., Durham, P. L. (2005). Sinus headache: A neurology, otolaryngology, allergy, and primary care consensus on diagnosis and treatment. *Mayo Clinic Proceedings, 80*(7), 908–916.

Causes of fibromyalgia remain a medical mystery. (2002, October 14). *Globe and Mail,* p. H1.

Ceccarelli, L. (2005). A hard look at ourselves: A reception study of rhetoric of science. *Technical Communication Quarterly, 14*(3), 257–265.

Chester, A. C. (2005). The demise of the sinus headache is premature. *Archives of Internal Medicine, 165*, 954.

Chow, R. (2010). The elusive material: What the dog doesn't understand. In D. Coole and S. Frost (Eds.), *New materialisms: Ontology, agency, and politics* (pp. 201–220). Durham, NC: Duke University Press.

Cicero, M. T. (1942). De partitione oratoria. In H. Rackham (Trans.), *Cicero in twenty-eight volumes: Volume IV* (pp. 306–421). Cambridge, MA: Harvard University Press.

Cicero, M. T. (1949). *De inventione.* (H. M. Hubbell, Trans.). Cambridge, MA: Harvard University Press.

Cleland, L. W. (2004). Modern bootlegging and the prohibition on fair prices: Last call for the repeal of pharmaceutical price gouging. *bepress Legal Series,* 264.

Cold, cough, allergy, bronchodilator, and antiasthmatic drug products for over-the-counter human use. 21 C.F.R. § 341 (2014).

Cold, cough, allergy, bronchodilator, and antiasthmatic drug products for over-the-counter human use; proposed amendment of the final monograph for over-the-counter nasal decongestant drug products. 69 Fed. Reg. 46119 (2004, 2 August) (to be codified at 21 C.F.R. pts. 310 and 431).

Cold, cough, allergy, bronchodilator, and antiasthmatic drug products for over-the-counter human use; amendment of the final monograph for over-the-counter nasal decongestant drug products. 70 Fed. Reg. 58974 (2005, 11 October) (to be codified at 21 C.F.R. pts. 310 and 431).

Collins, H. M., & Evans, R. (2002). The third wave of science studies: Studies of expertise and experience. *Social Studies of Science, 32*(2), 235–296.

Coole, D., & Frost, S. (2010). Introducing the new materialisms. In Coole and Frost (Eds.), *New materialisms: Ontology, agency, and politics* (pp. 1–43). Durham, NC: Duke University Press.

Coole, D. H. (2007). *Merleau-Ponty and modern politics after anti-humanism.* Lanham, MD: Rowman & Littlefield Publishers.

Cooper, R. M. (2006). The struggle for the 1906 act. In W. L. Pines (Ed.), *FDA: A century of consumer protection* (pp. 25–70). Washington, DC: Food and Drug Law Institute.

Crimes and criminal procedure. 18 U.S.C. §§ 208, 712.

Crofford, L. J., Rowbotham, M. C., Mease, P. J., Russell, I. J., Dworkin, R. H., Corbin, A. E., Young, J. P., LaMoreaux, L. K., Martin, S. A., & Sharma, U. (2005). Pregabalin for the treatment of fibromyalgia syndrome: Results of a randomized, double-blind, placebo-controlled trial. *Arthritis and Rheumatism, 52*(4), 1264–1273.

Crout, J. R., Vodra, W. W., & Werble, C. P. (2006). FDA's role in the pathway to safe and effective drugs. In W. L. Pines (Ed.), *FDA: A century of consumer protection* (pp. 159–194). Washington, DC: Food and Drug Law Institute.

DeNoon, D. J. (2003). Sinus headache symptoms = migraine? *WebMD Health News*, Retrieved 6 November, 2008, from http://www.webmd.com/migraines-headaches/news/20030318/sinus-headaches

Descartes, R. (1998). *Discourse on method and meditations on first philosophy.* (D. A. Cress, Trans.). Indianapolis: Hackett. (Original work published 1637)

Descartes, R. (2004). The treatise on man. In S. Gaukroger (Ed., Trans.). *The world and other writings* (pp. 99–169). Cambridge: Cambridge University Press.

Damjanov, I. (2006). *Pathology for the health professions.* Elsevier Health Sciences.

Dumit, J. (2004). *Picturing personhood: Brain scans and biomedical identity.* Princeton, NJ: Princeton University Press.

Dunn, G., & Everett, B. (1995). *Clinical biostatistics: An introduction to evidence-based medicine.* London: Edward Arnold.

Easton, C. F. (1897). *U.S. Patent No. 581199.* Washington, DC: U.S. Patent and Trademark Office.

Elliott, C. (2003). *Better than well: American medicine meets the American dream.* New York: W. W. Norton and Company.

Elliott, C. (2010). *White coat, black hat: Adventures on the dark side of medicine.* Boston: Beacon Press.

An encyclopaedia of medicine and surgery (1844). New York: C. H. Goodwin.

Engel, G. L. (1977). The need for a new medical model: A challenge for biomedicine. *Science, 196,* 129–136.

Engelhardt, H. T. (1976). Ideology and etiology. *Journal of Medicine and Philosophy, 1*(3), 256–268.

Eross, E., Dodick, D., & Eross, M. (2007). The sinus allergy and migraine study (SAMS). *Headache, 47*(2), 213–224.

FDA Center for Drug Evaluation and Research. (2007, June 21). Division Director Review and Basis for Approval Action. (Re: FDA Application Number 21–445/S-010. FOIA obtained.)

Fibromyalgia Network. (n.d.). Advocacy. Retrieved from http://www.fmnetnews.com/awareness/advocacy

Fishman, S., & Berger, L. (2000). *The war on pain.* New York: Quill.

Flexner, A. (1910). *Medical education in the United States and Canada: A report to the Carnegie Foundation for the Advancement of Teaching.* New York: The Carnegie Foundation.

Food and Drug Administration (FDA). (2003). Meeting of Arthritis Advisory Committee, Monday, June 23, 2003. [Transcript.] (FOIA obtained.)

Food and Drug Administration (FDA). (2007, June 21). Living with fibromyalgia: First drug approved. FDA Consumer Health Information. www.fda.gov/consumer/updates/fibromyalgia062107.html

Food and Drug Administration (FDA). (2008). *Guidance for the public, FDA Advisory Committee members, and FDA staff on procedures for determining conflict of interest and eligibility for participation in FDA Advisory Committees.* Retrieved August 2, 2013, from http://www.fda.gov/downloads/Regulatory Information/Guidances/UCM125646.pdf

Food and Drug Administration (FDA). (2009). Information for clinical investigators. http://www.fda.gov/Drugs/DevelopmentApprovalProcess/HowDrugs areDevelopedandApproved/ApprovalApplications/InvestigationalNewDrug INDApplication/ucm176259.htm

Food and Drug Administration (FDA). (2010, April 22). Patient Representative Program. Retrieved from http://www.fda.gov/forconsumers/byaudience/for patientadvocates/

Food and Drug Administration (FDA). (n.d.). How FDA reviews proposed drug names. Retrieved from http://www.fda.gov/downloads/Drugs/DrugSafety /MedicationErrors/UCM080867.pdf

Foucault, M. (1970). *The order of things: An archaeology of the human sciences.* New York: Vintage Books. (Original work published 1966)

Foucault, M. (1972). *The archaeology of knowledge and the discourse on language.* (A. M. S. Smith, Trans.). New York: Pantheon Books. (Original work published 1969)

Foucault, M. (1973). *The birth of the clinic.* (A. M. Sheridan, Trans.). Routledge: London. (Original work published 1963)

Fuller, S. (2006). *The philosophy of science and technology studies.* New York: Routledge.

Gad, C., & Jensen, C. (2010). On the consequences of post-ANT. *Science Technology and Human Values, 35*(1), 55–80.

Galen. (1976). *On the affected parts.* (R. E. Siegel, Trans.). New York: S. Karger.

Galison, P. (2008). Ten problems in history and philosophy of science. *Isis, 99,* 111–124.

Gaonkar, D. P. (1997). The idea of rhetoric in the rhetoric of science. In A. G. Gross & W. M. Keith (Eds.), *Rhetorical hermeneutics: Invention and interpretation the age of science* (pp. 25–85). Albany, NY: SUNY Press.

Gardner, P. (2003). Distorted packaging: Marketing depression as illness, drugs as cure. *Journal of Medical Humanities, 24*(1), 105–130.

Glickman, S. W., McHutchison, J. G., Peterson, E. D., Cairns, C. B., Harrington, R. A., Califf, R. M., & Schulman, K. A. (2009). Ethical and scientific implications of the globalization of clinical research. *New England Journal of Medicine, 360*(8), 816–823.

Goff, K. G. (2002, January 6). Getting a grip again: Pain medication, therapy relieve fibromyalgia. *Washington Times*, p. D1.

Gøtzsche, P. C., Hróbjartsson, A., Johansen, H. K., Haahr, M. T., Altman, D. G., & Chan, A. W. (2007). Ghost authorship in industry-initiated randomised trials. *PLoS Medicine, 4*(1), e19.

Grabill, J. (2006). The study of writing in the social factory: Methodology and rhetorical agency. In J. B. Scott, B. Longo, & K. V. Willis (Eds.), *Critical power tools* (pp. 151–170). Albany, NY: SUNY Press.

Graham, S. S. (2009). Agency and the rhetoric of medicine: Biomedical brain scans and the ontology of fibromyalgia. *Technical Communication Quarterly, 18*(4), 376–404.

Graham, S. S. (2011). Dis-ease or disease? Ontological rarefaction in the medical-industrial complex. *Journal of Medical Humanities, 32*(3), 167–187.

Graham, S. S., & Herndl, C. G. (2011). Talking off-label: A nonmodern science of pain in the medical-industrial complex. *Rhetoric Society Quarterly, 42*(2), 145–167.

Graham, S. S., & Herndl, C. G. (2013). Multiple ontologies in pain management: Towards a postplural rhetoric of science. *Technical Communication Quarterly, 22*(1), 103–125.

Griffing, G. T. (2008). Fibromyalgia is not a rheumatologic disease anymore. *Medscape Journal of Medicine, 10*(2), 47.

Gross, A. G. (1994). The role of rhetoric in the public understanding of science. *Public Understanding of Science, 3*(1), 3–23.

Gross, A. G. (2004). Why Hermagoras still matters: The fourth stasis and interdisciplinarity. *Rhetoric Review, 23*(2), 141–55.

Gross, A. G. (2005). Kuhn's incommensurability. In R. A. Harris (Ed.), *Rhetoric and incommensurability* (pp. 179–197). West Lafayette, IN: Parlor Press.

Grosz, E. (1994). *Volatile bodies: Toward a corporeal feminism.* Bloomington: Indiana University Press.

Grosz, E. (2010). Feminism, materialism, and freedom. In D. Coole and S. Frost (Eds.), *New materialisms: Ontology, agency, and politics* (pp. 139–157). Durham, NC: Duke University Press.

Haraway, D. J. (1997). *Modest_Witness@Second_Millennium.FemaleMan©_ Meets _OncoMouse™.* New York: Routledge.

Haraway, D. J. (1991). *Simians, cyborgs and women: The reinvention of nature.* New York: Routledge.

Harden, N. (2010). Objectification of the diagnostic criteria for CRPS. *Pain Medicine, 11*(8), 1212–1215.

Harman, G. (2009). *Prince of networks: Bruno Latour and metaphysics.* Melbourne, AU: re.press.

Harman, G. (2011). *The quadruple object.* Alresford, UK: John Hunt Publishing.

Harris, R. A. (2005). *Rhetoric and incommensurability.* West Lafayette, IN: Parlor Press.

Hauser, S. M., & Levine, H. L. (2008). Chronic daily headache: When to suspect sinus disease. *Current Pain and Headache Report, 12*(1), 45.

Healy, D. (2004). *The creation of psychopharmacology.* Cambridge, MA: Harvard University Press.

Heidegger, M. (1971). The thing. In *Poetry, language, and thought* (pp. 165–186). New York: Harper & Row.

Heidegger, M. (2008). *Being and time.* New York: Harper & Row.

Heidlebaugh, N. J. (2001). *Judgment, rhetoric, and the problem of incommensurability: Recalling practical wisdom.* Columbia: University South Carolina Press.

Herndl, C. G. (1991). Writing ethnography: Representation, rhetoric, and institutional practices. *College English, 53*(3), 320–332.

Herndl, C. G. (2002). Rhetoric of science as non-modern practice. In F. Antczak, C. Coggins & G. Klinger (Eds.), *Professing rhetoric: Selected papers from the 2000 Rhetoric Society of America conference* (pp. 215–222). Mahwah, NJ: Lawrence Erlbaum.

Herndl, C. G., & Brown, S. C. (1996). *Green culture: Environmental rhetoric in contemporary America.* Madison I: University of Wisconsin Press.

Herndl, C. G., Fennel, B. A., & Miller, C. R. (1991). Understanding failures in organizational discourse: The accident at Three Mile Island and the shuttle *Challenger* disaster. In C. Bazerman & J. Paradis (Eds.), *Textual dynamics of the professions* (pp. 279–305). Madison: University of Wisconsin Press.

Hinton, J. (1914). *The mystery of pain: A book for the sorrowful.* New York: Mitchell Kennerly. (Original work published 1866)

Hippocrates. (1979). *Hippocrates with an English translation by W. H. S. Jones* (six-volume set). (W. H. S. Jones, Trans.). Cambridge, MA: Harvard University Press.

Holm, S., & Jonas, M. F. (Eds.). (2004). *Engaging the world: The use of empirical research in bioethics and the regulation of biotechnology.* Amsterdam: IOS Press.

Hounsfield, G. N. (1973a). Computerized transverse axial scanning (tomography): Part I: Description of system. *British Journal of Radiology, 46*, 1016–1022.

Hounsfield, G. N. (1973b). *U.S. Patent No. 3778614.* Washington, DC: U.S. Patent and Trademark Office.

Hulley, S. B. Cummings, S. R., Browner, W. S., Grady, D. G., & Newman, T. B. (2013). *Designing clinical research.* Philadelphia: Lippincott, Williams & Wilkins.

Hutson, S. (2009). Publication of fake journals raises ethical questions. *Nature Medicine, 15*(6), 598.

IASP Taskforce on Taxonomy. (1994). IASP pain terminology (International Association for the Study of Pain). Retrieved from http://www.iasp-pain.org

Institute of Medicine (IOM). (2009). *Conflict of interest in medical research, education, and practice.* Washington, DC: The National Academies Press.

Ishkanian, G., Blumenthal, H., Webster, C. J., Richardson, M. S., & Ames, M. (2007). Efficacy of sumatriptan tablets in migraineurs self-described or physician-diagnosed as having sinus headache: A randomized, double-blind, placebo-controlled study. *Clinical Therapeutics, 29*(1), 99–109.

Issuance of Multiple Prescriptions for Schedule II Controlled Substances, 72 Fed. Reg. 64921 (2007, 19 November) (to be codified at 21 C.F.R. pt. 1306).

Ives, J. (2008). "Encounters with experience": Empirical bioethics and the future. *Health Care Analysis, 16*(1), 1–6.

Ives, J., & Draper, H. (2009). Appropriate methodologies for empirical bioethics: It's all relative. *Bioethics, 23*(4), 249–258.

Jack, J. (2010). Object lessons: Recent work in rhetoric of science. *Quarterly Journal of Speech, 96*(2), 209–216.

Jack, J. L., & Appelbaum, G. (2010). "This is your brain on rhetoric": Research-directions for neurorhetorics. *Rhetoric Society Quarterly, 40*(5), 411–437.

Keith, W. M., & Beard, D. E. (2008). Toulmin's rhetorical logic: What's the warrant for warrants? *Philosophy and Rhetoric, 41*(1), 22–50.

Kennedy, G. A. (1983). *Greek rhetoric under the Christian emperors*. Princeton, NJ: Princeton University Press.

Keränen, L. (2010). *Scientific characters: Rhetoric, politics, and trust in breast cancer research*. Tuscaloosa: University of Alabama Press.

Kinirons, H., & Ellis, H. (2005). *French's index of differential diagnosis*. London: Hodder Arnold.

Kinsella, W. J. (2005). Rhetoric, action, and agency in institutionalized science and technology. *Technical Communication Quarterly, 14*(3), 303–310.

Klassen, P. E. (2001). *Blessed events: Religion and home birth in America*. Princeton, NJ: Princeton University Press.

Koerber, A. (1997). From folklore to fact: The rhetorical history of breastfeeding and immunity, 1950–1997. *Journal of Medical Humanities, 27*, 151–166.

Koerber, A. (2006a). Rhetorical agency, resistance, and the disciplinary rhetorics of breastfeeding. *Technical Communication Quarterly, 15*(1), 87–101.

Koerber, A. (2006b). From "Wives' tales and folklore" to scientific fact: Rhetorics of breastfeeding and immunity, 1950–1997. *Journal of Medical Humanities, 27*(3), 151–166.

Kuhn, T. S. (1996). *The structure of scientific revolutions* (3rd ed.). Chicago: University of Chicago Press.

Kumar, V., Abbas, A., & Fausto, N. (2005). *Robbins and Cotran pathologic basis of disease* (7th ed.). Philadelphia: Elsevier.

Latour, B. (1987). *Science in action: How to follow scientists and engineers through society*. Cambridge, MA: Harvard University Press.

Latour, B. (1991). *We have never been modern*. (C. Porter, Trans.). Cambridge, MA: Harvard University Press.

Latour, B. (1993). *The pasteurization of France*. Cambridge, MA: Harvard University Press.

Latour, B. (1999). *Pandora's hope: Essays on the reality of science studies*. Cambridge, MA: Harvard University Press.

Latour, B. (2004). Why has critique run out of steam? From matters of fact to matters of concern. *Critical Inquiry, 30*(2), 225–248.

Latour, B. (2005). *Reassembling the social: An introduction to actor-network theory*. Oxford: Oxford University Press.

Law, J. (1994). *Organizing modernity: Social ordering and social theory*. Hoboken, NJ: Wiley-Blackwell.

Leriche, R. (1939). *The surgery of pain*. Philadelphia: Williams & Wilkins.

Lewis, B. E. (2003). Prozac and the post-human politics of cyborgs. *Journal of Medical Humanities, 24*(1), 49–63.

Liebeskind, J. C., & Paul, L. A. (1977). Psychological and physiological mechanisms of pain. *Annual Review of Psychology, 28*, 41–60.

Liem, E. B., Joiner, T. V., Tsueda, K., & Sessler, D. I. (2005). Increased sensitivity to thermal pain and reduced subcutaneous lidocaine efficacy in redheads. *Anesthesiology, 102*(3), 509.

Lynch, J. A. (2009). Articulating scientific practice: Understanding Dean Hamer's "gay gene" study as overlapping material, social, and rhetorical registers. *Quarterly Journal of Speech, 95*(4), 435–456.

Keller, E. F. (1996). *Refiguring life: Metaphors of twentieth-century biology*. New York: Columbia University Press.

Marback, R. (2008). Unclenching the fist: Embodying rhetoric and giving objects their due. *Rhetoric Society Quarterly, 38*(1), 46–65.

McBride, P. (1900). *Diseases of the throat, nose, and ear: A clinical manual for students and practitioners*. Philadelphia: P. Blakiston's Son & Co. (Original work published 1891)

McCullough, M. (2000, November 6). Pain that often defines diagnosis. *Philadelphia Inquirer*, p. D01.

McDaniel, S. H., Hepworth, J., & Doherty, W. J. (1992). *Medical family therapy: A biopsychosocial approach to families with health problems*. New York: Basic Books.

McGee, Steven. (2007). *Evidence-based physical diagnosis*. St. Louis: Saunders/ Elsevier.

McKeon, R. (1966). The methods of rhetoric and philosophy: Invention and judgment. In L. Wallach (Ed.), *The classical tradition: Literary and historical essays in honor of Harry Caplan* (pp. 365–373). Ithaca, NY: Cornell University Press.

McKeon, R. (1987). *Rhetoric: Essays in invention and discovery*. M. Backman (Ed.). Woodbridge CT: Ox Bow Press.

Mehle, M. E., & Kremer, P. S. (2008). Sinus CT scan findings in "sinus headache" migraineurs. *Headache, 48*, 67–71.

Mehle, M. E., & Schreiber, C. P. (2005). Sinus headache, migraine, and the otolaryngologist. *Otolaryngology—Head and Neck Surgery, 133*, 489–496.

Melzack, R. (1973). *The puzzle of pain*. New York: Basic Books.

Melzack, R. (1975). The McGill pain questionnaire. Retrieved from http://www.ama-cmeonline.com/pain_mgmt/pdf/mcgill.pdf

Melzack, R., & Wall, P. D. (1982). *The challenge of pain*. London: Penguin.

MidAmerican Neuroscience Institute (n.d.). So you think you have a sinus headache? MidAmerican Neuroscience Institute. http://www.neurokc.com/mani2.aspx?pgID=990 (accessed April 12, 2011; no longer online).

Mol, A. (1999). Ontological politics. A word and some questions. In J. Law & J. Hassard (Eds.), *Actor network theory and after* (pp. 74–89). Oxford: Blackwell.

Mol, A. (2002). *The body multiple: Ontology in medical practice.* Durham, NC: Duke University Press.

Morris, D. B. (1991). *The culture of pain.* Berkeley: University of California Press.

Mould, R. F. (1993). *A century of X-rays and radioactivity in medicine with emphasis on photographic records of the early years.* Philadelphia: Institute of Physics Publishing.

Moynihan, R. (2009). Merck defends Vioxx in court, as publisher apologises for fake journal. *BMJ, 338,* b1914.

Moynihan, R., Heath, I., & Henry, D. (2002). Selling sickness: The pharmaceutical industry and disease mongering. *BMJ: British Medical Journal, 324*(7342), 886.

Moynihan, R., & Henry, D. (2006). The fight against disease mongering: Generating knowledge for action. *PLoS Medicine, 3*(4), e191.

Mudry, J. J. (2009). *Measured meals: Nutrition in America.* Albany, NY: SUNY Press.

National Headache Foundation. (2008). The complete guide to headache. Retrieved November 6, 2008, from http://www.headaches.org/educational_modules/competeguide

Neuner, R. (2007). Clinical review. (Re: FDA Application Number 21–445/S-010. FOIA obtained.)

Ophir, D., Gross-Isseroff, R., Lancet, D., & Marshak, G. (1986). Changes in olfactory acuity by total inferior turbinectomy. *JAMA Head and Neck Surgery, 112*(2), 195–197.

Perrot, S., Dickenson, A. H., & Bennett, R. M. (2008). Fibromyalgia: Harmonizing science with clinical practice considerations. *Pain Practice: World Institute of Pain Proceedings,* 1–13.

Petryna, A. (2009). *When experiments travel: Clinical trials and the global search for human subjects.* Princeton, NJ: Princeton University Press.

Pharmacy update—Fibromyalgia: Treating the enigma. (2007, December 22). *Chemist and Druggist,* p. 17.

Pickering, A. (1995). *The mangle of practice: Time, agency, and science.* Chicago: University of Chicago Press.

Pickering, A. (2010). *The cybernetic brain: Sketches of another future.* Chicago: University of Chicago Press.

Ploeger, J. S. (2009). *The boundaries of the new frontier: Rhetoric and communication at Fermi National Accelerator Laboratory.* Columbia: University of South Carolina Press.

Prelli, L. J. (2005). Stasis and the problem of incommensurate communication: The case of spousal violence research. In R.A. Harris (Ed.), *Rhetoric and incommensurability* (pp. 294–331). West Lafayette, IN: Parlor Press.

Quinter, J. L., & Cohen, M. L. (1999). Fibromyalgia falls foul of fallacy. *The Lancet, 353*(9), 1092.

Resnik, D. B., Rehm, M., & Minard, R. (2001). The undertreatment of pain:

Scientific, clinical, cultural, and philosophical factors. *Medicine, Health Care, and Philosophy, 4*(3), 277–288.

Rey, R. (1993). *The history of pain.* (L. E. Wallace, J. A. Cadden, & S. W. Cadden, Trans.). Cambridge, MA: Harvard University Press.

Rey, R. (1995). *The history of pain* (part 2). J. A. Cadden & S. W. Cadden (Eds.). Cambridge, MA: Harvard University Press.

Rheinberger, H. J. (2010). *Epistemology of the concrete.* Durham, NC: Duke University Press.

Richards, I. A. (1936). *The philosophy of rhetoric.* New York: Oxford University Press.

Rickert, T. (2013). *Ambient rhetoric: The attunements of rhetorical being.* Pittsburgh: University of Pittsburgh Press.

Roland, P. E. (1985). Applications of brain blood flow imaging in behavioral neurophysiology: Cortical field activation hypothesis. In L. Sokoloff (Ed.), *Brain imaging and brain function* (87–104). New York: Raven Press.

Rose, G. (2001). *Visual methodologies: An introduction to the interpretation of visual materials.* London: Sage.

Rose, N. (2006). Disorders without borders? The expanding scope of psychiatric practice. *BioSocieties, 1*(4), 465.

Scott, J. B. (2003). Extending rhetorical-cultural analysis: Transformations of home HIV testing. *College English, 65*(4), 349–367.

Scott, J. B. (2004). Tracking rapid HIV testing through the cultural circuit: Implications for technical communication. *Journal of Business and Technical Communication, 18*(2), 198–219.

Scott, W. R., Ruef, M., Mendel, P., & Caronna, C. (2000). *Institutional change and health care organizations: From professional dominance to managed care.* Chicago: University of Chicago Press.

Segal, J. (2005). *Health and the rhetoric of medicine.* Carbondale: Southern Illinois University Press.

Shannon, C. E., & Weaver, W. (1949). *The mathematical theory of communication.* Urbana: University of Illinois Press.

Shapin, S., & Shaffer, S. (1985). *Leviathan and the air-pump: Hobbes, Boyle, and the experimental life.* Princeton, NJ: Princeton University Press.

Shea, E. P. (2008). *How the gene got its groove.* Albany, NY: SUNY Press.

Sherrington, C. S. (1903). Qualitative differences of spinal reflex corresponding with qualitative difference of cutaneous stimulus. *Journal of Physiology, 30*, 39–46.

Sherrington, C. S. (1906). *The integrative action of the nervous system.* New Haven, CT: Yale University Press.

Shim, C., & Williams, H. (1983). Relationship of wheezing to the severity of obstruction in asthma. *JAMA Internal Medicine, 143*(5), 890–892.

Shir, Y., & Fitzcharles, M. (2009). Should rheumatologists retain ownership of fibromyalgia? *Journal of Rheumatology. 26*(4), 667–670.

Shulman, L., Pretzer-Aboff, I., Anderson, K.E., Sevenson, R., Vaughn, C.G., Gruber-Baldini, A.L., Reich, S.G., & Weiner, W.J. (2006). Subjective report versus objective measurement of activities of daily living in Parkinson's disease. *Movement Disorders, 21*(6), 794–799.

Sismondo, S. (2007). Ghost management: How much of the medical literature is shaped behind the scenes by the pharmaceutical industry? *PLoS Medicine, 4*(9), e286.

Spivak, G. C. (1999). *A critique of postcolonial reason: Toward a history of the vanishing present.* Cambridge, MA: Harvard University Press.

Star, S. L. (1995). *Ecologies of knowledge: Work and politics in science and technology.* Albany: State University of New York Press.

Star, S. L., & Griesemer, J. (1989). Institutional ecology, "translations" and boundary objects: Amateurs and professionals in Berkeley's Museum of Vertebrate Zoology. *Social Studies of Science, 19*, 387–420.

Starr, P. (1982). *The social transformation of American medicine.* New York: Basic Books.

Stevens, R. (1999). The complexity of pain: No pain without gain: The augmentation of nociception in the CNS. *Physical Therapy Reviews, 4*(2), 105–116.

Ter-Pogossian, M.M. (1979). *U.S. Patent No. 4150292.* Washington, DC: U.S. Patent and Trademark Office.

Ter-Pogossian, M. M., Phelps, M. E., Hoffman, E. J., & Mullani, N. A. (1975). A positron-emission transaxial tomography for nuclear imaging (PETT). *Radiology, 114*, 89–98.

Teston, C. B., & Graham, S. S. (2012). Stasis theory and meaningful public participation in pharmaceutical policy-making. *Present Tense: A Journal of Rhetoric in Society, 2*(2). Retrieved from http://www.presenttensejournal.org/volume-2/stasis-theory-and-meaningful-public-participation-in-pharmaceutical-policy-making/

Teston, C., Graham, S. S., Baldwinson, R., Li, A., Swift, J. (2014). Public voices in pharmaceuticals deliberations: Negotiating "clinical benefit" in FDA's Avastin hearing. *Journal of Medical Humanities, 35*, 149–170.

Thévenot, L. (2002). Which road to follow? The moral complexity of an "equipped" humanities. In J. Law & A. Mol (Eds.), *Complexities: Social studies of knowledge practices* (pp. 53–87). Durham, NC: Duke University Press.

Thomson, E. (1897). *U.S. Patent No. 583956.* Washington, DC: U.S. Patent and Trademark Office.

Toulmin, S. E. (2003). *The uses of argument.* Cambridge: Cambridge University Press. (Original work published 1958)

Turner, J. A., Deyo, R. A., Loeser, J. D., Von Korff, M., & Fordyce, W. E. (1994). The importance of placebo effects in pain treatment and research. *JAMA, 271*(20), 1609–1614.

Turner, S. P. (1990). Forms of patronage. In S. E. Cozzens & T. S. Gieryn (Eds.),

Theories of science in society (pp. 185–211). Bloomington: Indiana University Press.

Underwood, A. (2003, May 19). Fibromyalgia: Not all in your head. *Newsweek*, p. 53.

U.S. Department of Health and Human Services, Food and Drug Administration, Center for Drug Evaluation and Research (CDER), Center for Biologics Evaluation and Research (CBER) & Center for Veterinary Medicine (CVM). (January 2012). *Guidance for Industry: Product Name Placement, Size, and Prominence in Advertising and Promotional Labeling.* Retrieved from http://www.fda.gov/downloads/Drugs/.../Guidances/ucm070076.pdf

Waddell, C. (1990). The role of pathos in the decision-making process: A study in the rhetoric of science policy. In R. A. Harris (Ed.), *Landmark essays on rhetoric of science: Case studies* (pp. 127–150). Mahwah, NJ: Hermagoras Press.

Wade, C. H. (1897). Wanted, a name—"electrography." *British Medical Journal*, 2 (1905), 52.

Waldeyer, W. (1891). *Ueber einige neure forschungen im gebiete der anatomie des centralnervensystems.* Leipzig: Georg Thieme.

Walker, J. (2000). *Rhetoric and poetics in antiquity.* Oxford: Oxford University Press.

Walzer, A. E., & Gross, A. (1994). Positivists, postmodernists, Aristotelians and the *Challenger* disaster. *College English, 56*, 420–433.

Whitbeck, C. (1981). What is diagnosis? Some critical reflections. *Theoretical Medicine and Bioethics 2*(3), 319–329.

WHO Scientific Group. (1975). *Guidelines for evaluation of drugs for use in man.* Geneva: World Health Organization.

Williams, D., & Gracely, R. H. (2006). Functional magnetic resonance imaging findings in fibromyalgia. *Arthritis Research and Therapy, 8*, 224–232.

Williams, S. J., Martin, P., & Gabe, J. (2011). The pharmaceuticalisation of society? A framework for analysis. *Sociology of Health & Illness, 33*(5), 710–725.

Wilson, G., & Herndl, C. G. (2007). Boundary objects as rhetorical exigence: Knowledge mapping and multidisciplinary cooperation at the Los Alamos National Laboratory. *Journal of Business and Technical Communication, 21*(2), 129–154.

Wisberg, D. S., Keil, F. C., Goodstein, J., Rawson, E., & Gray, J. R. (2008). The seductive allure of neuroscience explanations. *Journal of Cognitive Neuroscience, 20*(3), 470–477.

Wolinsky, H. (2005). Disease mongering and drug marketing. *EMBO reports, 6*(7), 612.

Woloshin, S., & Schwartz, L. M. (2006). Giving legs to restless legs: A case study of how the media helps make people sick. *PLoS Medicine, 3*(4), e170.

Zatzick, D. F., & Dimsdale, J. E. (1990). Cultural variations in response to painful stimuli. *Psychosomatic Medicine, 52*(5), 544–557.

Index